AGROUND!

AGROUND!

Coping with Emergency Groundings

BY JAMES E. MINNOCH

Illustrations by Jim Sollers

Distributed by:
Airlife Publishing Ltd.
101 Longden Road, Shrewsbury SY3 9EB, England

For Sarah,
who sailed away on the great
uncharted oceans of life

Library of Congress Catalog Card No. 85-71609
ISBN Number 0-8286-0098-8

John de Graff Inc.
Clinton Corners, N.Y. 12514

Printed in U.S.A.

ACKNOWLEDGMENTS

Special thanks to
Stuart, John, Hal, and Boh
for their cooperation and trust.

Contents

PART THREE
PRECARIOUS GROUNDINGS

PART FOUR
GROUNDING CASES

APPENDICES

Introduction

Today we can use satellites for pinpoint navigational accuracy, our boats have evolved to use superstrong and durable materials, and a vast knowledge of seamanship is duly recorded. Yet, after thousands of years of sailing history, we have not devoted an adequate amount of research engineering effort to the important aspect of extricating boats gone aground—a problem acknowledged to be of predominant concern to yachtsmen the world over. Every small-boat sailor should have a working knowledge of how to handle a grounding, and this book is designed to stimulate continuing efforts to devise new methods and techniques for coping with these always shocking and sometimes disastrous situations.

It was not my deliberate intention to become a writer on small-boat groundings; it just evolved. Several years ago I wrote a magazine article about a lay-over type of grounding that I experienced in *Springtide,* our 33-foot Bristol sloop, citing lessons to be learned. There was such great interest in the subject that I then extended my research for articles in several other yachting magazines, which, in turn, generated additional widespread interest. My research into this unhappy subject became quite extensive as virtually every aspect of many case studies was examined, from normal kedging-off to the extreme of abandoning a vessel without hope. The subject is intriguing and potentially of great value to yachtsmen.

The groundings I experienced were of interest to others because I normally cruise under some of the worst conditions found anywhere in the United States: from Mount Desert Island, Maine, north to Canada in the perpetually cold North Atlantic. Here prevail the greatest tides (to 30 feet at Eastport, Maine) and the stormiest conditions in the nation. This rocky, boulder-strewn coast is also the foggiest place in the United States, contributing to the natural fear of going aground with the possible loss of the yacht and extreme danger to crew-members. Nevertheless, there is no place I would rather cruise. So, rather than abandon the adventure of cruising these "worst-case" waters, we have devised courses of action to help cope with the inevitable groundings.

Experience is the great teacher in boathandling, so I have drawn from the experiences of many other skippers, some of them distin-guished contemporary mariners, and others who have sailed off before us. The theoretical approach and the proven practical approaches stand side by side for you, the reader, to evaluate. And evaluate you must, for each experience is unique.

Anyone can go aground—sometimes euphemistically called *being stuck.* Perhaps the most newsworthy simple grounding in modern times occurred on May 3, 1983, when the 75,700-ton nuclear-powered aircraft carrier U.S.S. *Enterprise* went aground in San Francisco Bay. The 1,123-foot-long ship had slipped out of the 42-foot-deep channel and slid to an ignoble stop in 29 feet of water, a mere 1,700 yards from the end of a 46,500-mile voyage. Three thousand friends and relatives waited in frustration for five hours at Alameda Naval Air Station while the captain worked to extricate the mammoth vessel.

The U.S. Navy, with all its vast resources, was unable to free the ship. Many usual techniques were employed. Eleven tugs tried to budge *Enterprise,* pushing and towing, but to no avail. Then the 3,500-man crew was assembled on the port deck, and water was shifted in the ballast tanks—all this to heel the ship in hopes of freeing her. But the keel, which normally requires 36 feet of water for safe clearance, remained stuck. Only with the help of the tide did the *Enterprise* finally break loose from her unwanted mooring and finish her long journey home. The accident was mostly an embarrassment, but it demon-strates that groundings can happen to the best of skippers, from those commanding the largest of ships to those navigating the smallest pleasure boat.

Moreover, insurance statistics reveal that virtually the same number of grounding claims are placed by sailors with advanced train-ing as novice sailors with no training—as opposed to other loss categories where trained and experienced sailors file far fewer claims.

Sailboats are faced with a special set of conditions in extricating themselves when they are aground. The configurations of sailboat keels can complicate groundings, sometimes putting a boat over on its topsides as the tide recedes. Usually, low-powered auxiliary engines cannot develop the thrust to drag the keel off in order to unground, or refloat, the boat. And the centers of gravity and buoyancy can place weight where it is least needed in a grounding situation. On the other hand, an initial grounding may be simpler with a sailboat than with other hull types because of the reduced area in contact with the bottom. Sailboats may also be tilted more readily to free the keel. Each grounding has its own distinct conditions, is unique in its own way.

The techniques described herein for freeing a grounded sailboat have been used successfully over the years. Such techniques usually entail a combination of the knowledgeable utilization of the art and science of good seamanship and being prepared with the proper equipment, or being able to improvise adequately. Because each situation is an accident, it requires a realistic evaluation of the situation, knowledge of accepted techniques, imagination in applying techniques with the tools and assistance available—and luck.

Thus, the methods suggested here will often need to be used in varying combinations to be effective. Examine the full range of choices. Experiment until you discover a solution. The chances of salvaging a boat even from hard groundings are quite good when compared to the similar plight of sailing ships, which almost always were lost.

The state of the art of refloating a grounded small vessel changes slowly but continuously. Every experienced yachtsman has valuable experiences and opinions that will round out the information presented here. Meanwhile, I am hopeful that this book will be helpful in alleviating one of the greatest fears associated with yachting—that of going aground.

PART ONE

BASIC KNOWLEDGE

CHAPTER 1

Be Prepared: Boat and Gear

In order to be totally prepared for any emergency, your first rule must be to know your boat or the one on which you are sailing. Of special importance in every grounding situation is your knowledge of your boat's underwater configuration, including the shapes of the bilge, keel, and rudder. Know how she is usually loaded. Know what you can expect from your engine. Review the list of equipment you will need for a grounding.

Bilge Shape and Stability

The term *bilge* refers to the part of the hull where it turns out and upward from the keel below the waterline (the term also relates to the area inside the hull where bilge water collects). Sailors have great interest in the shape of the bilges, since their shape determines, to a significant degree, how stiff or how tender a boat will be. A boat with steep or slack bilges with considerable deadrise will be tender and will depend on ballast to maintain stability. A boat with round bilges, on the other hand, may be quite subject to rolling, the hull having a lack of bearing with no "shoulders" to supply natural stability. Nevertheless, virtually every sailboat is designed to dry out (when laid over with a falling tide) on her bilges without taking water in the cockpit.

Keel Shape

Knowing the keel configuration of your boat is important in a grounding, since that helps determine your approach to getting your boat off (or, in Coast Guard terminology, *ungrounding the boat*). Keels come in many shapes, of course, but the most common ones are full length, modified full-length, fin, and centerboard keels. Except for boats with centerboard keels, there is a designed forefoot from the bowstem to the bottom of the keel—an angle of 60 percent for full-keeled hulls to 44 percent on certain modified keels. These architectural specifications relate to the boat's sailing performance but also are of interest to the skipper of a grounded boat. Because of the forefoot, the lowest part of the forward point on a full-length keel, for example, usually is just abaft the mast step and runs in a straight line aft to the sternpost. Thus, it is even possible that the weight of crewmembers on the point of the bow would tip the bow down enough to allow the boat to be pulled off aft—assuming, of course, that the keel is grounded on its forward lowest point.

In order to understand the configuration of the keel on my boat, a Bristol 33-foot (10-meter) sloop with a modified full keel, I took several photographs of the bottom, at a perpendicular angle, when she was hauled on a railway. I keep these photographs in the boat's log so that I can refer to them easily when needed, such as when the boat is hauled by a TraveLift and the operator needs to know where to position the straps. I also transferred the locations of the essential keel and rudder measurements to points on the deck, and made a record of them in the log. Thus, the deepest point of the aft part of the keel is six inches forward of the genoa winches, the deepest point of the forward section of the keel is directly below the forward lower spreader chainplate, and so forth. When aground, I have reference points from which to work. (Over-the-side lead soundings also can sometimes tell me the point at which I'm aground and indicate which direction the keel needs to be shifted.)

The Rudder

It is just as important that you know the location and shape of your boat's rudder. All sailboat rudders have some clearance above the lowest point of the keel, even if it is only the width of a skeg. Pulling a boat off by the stern, for example, can demolish a rudder if it is forced into the ground or into some other obstacle. There have been cases where the rudder alone has held a boat aground. If you know the rudder's exact location and shape, you will be better able to determine the direction in which the boat should be pulled free, thus avoiding rocks and other obstructions. This knowledge will also come in handy in other situations, such as when you are drying out the hull and need to ensure protection for the rudder.

Adequate Ground Tackle

It seems that you never can have too much ground tackle. Anchors and a lot of line are needed in most groundings, the quantity depending on the situation. A heavy anchor is needed for a kedge, other anchors to stabilize or secure a grounded boat from moving about on the bottom. Often two kedges work better than one. You usually will need long kedge and shore lines, so have aboard plenty of extra heavy line. This is a time when line with low stretch under strain, such as Dacron, is better than nylon line that will elongate over more than one-fourth of its length when under great strain. (See Appendix A for a table of rope-breaking strengths.)

Carry a minimum of two anchors—one heavy storm anchor and a normal working anchor. Anchor lines, or rodes, should be on the stout side, since enormous strains will be placed on them. Carry a minimum of three 300-foot kedge lines—one for each anchor and one spare length.

I carry—and use—five anchors for our 33-foot sloop: a 44-pound Bruce (bow anchor), two 22-pound Danforths, one 25-pound wishbone, and one 35-pound fisherman/yachtsman. Each has a rode. Two are ⅝-inch nylon and three are ½-inch nylon. I also carry about 200 feet of spare ⁹⁄₁₆-inch Dacron sheet and halyard line that can be used for kedging. The anchors all have 15 feet of ⅜-inch chain leaders, with the exception of the working bow anchor, which carries 20 feet of ½-inch chain.

All this may sound like overkill, but there are times when I have had to use it all—and stripped the standing halyards and sheets besides. When drying out a boat (see Chapter 12), it is not uncommon to have two kedges out and two or three anchors or shore lines belayed to secure the boat. Often you can run lines to docks, rocks, or trees some distance away if you have enough. Most long-range-cruising sailors carry a large inventory of ground tackle, not just to be able to cope with different anchoring situations but also to be more self-sufficient in dealing with the inevitable groundings.

Sounding Lead

In selecting the direction for refloating, you will need some way of determining the depth of the water around your grounded boat. (See Figure 1.) This is normally done from a dinghy with a sounding lead and measured line. You can also take soundings from the deck, but this may be insufficient to provide information on a clear channel to follow. If you do not have a sounding lead, you can fabricate one from a heavy weight (one to five pounds) and a length of low-stretch Dacron line. Be sure to measure and mark the line carefully while it is under strain in order to obtain accurate readings of water depth. Take soundings by bouncing the weight on the bottom until you are confident you

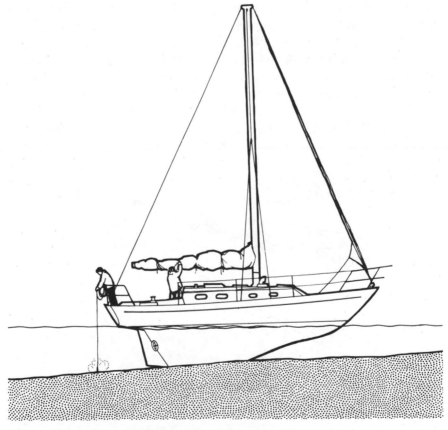

Figure 1. Verify the direction of deeper water with leadline soundings. Take the soundings from the deck, as shown here, or use a dinghy, recording depths at locations all around the grounded boat.

can obtain a true reading from the measuring marks on the line. Plot these soundings in relation to the location of the boat, and save the plotting sheet for reference. I carry several plastic jugs and small buoys to which I tie light line or string and weights to mark a channel for indicating the direction in which the boat should most favorably be refloated. Remember that the bottom contour may be irregular and you could go aground more than once. Inches of water can be critical in successful ungroundings.

Handybilly

The handybilly is simply a portable block-and-tackle arrangement that can be useful for refloating tasks. (See Figure 2.) It is similar to the common boom vang, but normally it is composed of heavier materials, i.e., larger blocks and thicker line. In a grounding, the handybilly provides extra pulling power when it is attached to a kedge line. Sailing ships and most older sailboats always carried this device for many heavy pulling or lifting chores, but powerful modern sailboat winches have reduced the need for it. Nevertheless, it is a versatile tool for dealing with the endless variations to grounding situations where extra pull is needed.

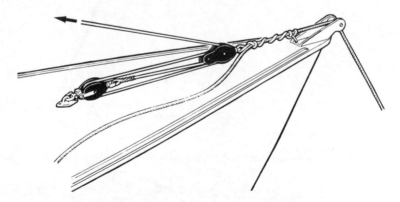

Figure 2. A handybilly rigged from secure fittings will place additional strain on a kedge line.

The mechanical advantage of any purchase is the number of parts to the running block (as opposed to the standing block). The safe working load (SWL) in tons of purchase (making an allowance for sheave friction or resistance in the tackle) is:

$$SWL = \frac{(10)(MA)(SWL_{line})}{(10 + N)},$$

where MA = mechanical advantage of purchase
SWL_{line} = safe working load (in tons) of the line rove in the purchase
N = number of sheaves in the system.

To calculate the pull necessary to lift a known weight (P) with a purchase, use:

$$P = \frac{W + [(0.1)(W)(N)]}{10 + N},$$

where W = load weight
N = number of sheaves in the system
MA = mechanical advantage of purchase.

Blocks

A well-equipped yacht always carries extra blocks, not only as spares for running rigging but also for routing lines to winches and cleats. For example, most sailors know that they can rig blocks in order to angle docking lines to a favored direction. Seldom, however, do sailors use the same technique to route anchor, or kedge, lines to advantageous points aboard the boat. Stout blocks can be used to direct a kedge line to the most powerful winch on the boat (often a hydraulic or electric anchor winch at the bow) even if the line must be routed the entire length of the boat. Blocks are also useful when careening the boat with the use of an anchor (see Shifting the Keel), whereby a halyard is rove through a block belayed to an anchor line. Snatchblocks are preferable because they can be opened to receive the line.

Deck Hardware

Many sailors do not realize the tremendous strain and torque imposed on deck fixtures used in conjunction with towing, pulling, or stabilizing a grounded boat. Deck hardware must be bolted through large, strong backing plates. This includes cleats, winches, chocks, and fairleads. The fixtures must be of the proper size to accept the larger lines that are used frequently in groundings—say, for example, ¾-inch towlines. Never use undersized or improperly installed hardware. It can cause injury when it breaks free while under heavy strain. (More on this subject appears in Chapter 10.)

Planning to Lighten Your Vessel

Develop a plan to lighten your boat to add buoyancy for refloating. Sufficient reduction of displacement, through the removal of weight, allows the boat to float higher. Figure out a way to drain all tanks and pump the liquid overboard (special valves can be installed for this purpose, with the bilge pump doing the pumping). Prepare a list of items that can be removed and placed in other boats or taken ashore to lighten the boat and protect valuable equipment. It is possible at dockside to obtain an estimate of how weight loaded on your boat affects your waterline. This should be recorded for future use. Thus, by placing known weight aboard or removing it from a specific boat, the skipper will be able to gain some insight into the effect of removing weight in a grounding situation. A lighter boat is also more easily towed off the bottom. (See Chapter 3 for additional information on this.)

Flashlight

In case of night groundings, each crewmember should carry a small personal flashlight on a lanyard. I also attach a whistle. You will need one or more portable spotlights, preferably ones that are wired to the ship's 12-volt power system. It seems that you can never have enough good flashlights. The best type of portable flashlight uses a 6-volt battery that should be good for an entire season. I carry three of these, in addition to five D-battery-size hand flashlights. I also keep on board a good supply of replacement batteries and bulbs, which are properly protected from moisture. Rechargeable nickel-cadmium batteries will do well if you replace them about every two or three weeks with freshly charged batteries. I find that the 6-volt rechargeable batteries (available from Sears) will last an entire season with limited use. There are several good brands of waterproof flashlights on the market today. Buy the best and you will not be sorry.

CHAPTER 2

Be Prepared: Handling the Crew

As the skipper of a grounded boat, you should be prepared for a variety of psychological reactions from the crew—everything from festive hilarity to outright shock. You must maintain a high degree of self-control, remaining calm, calculating, and in command throughout the grounding incident. And you should concentrate on the problem at hand, setting aside your own emotions.

All groundings can have detrimental psychological effects on crewmembers. These may not necessarily entail fear or doubt, but perhaps a bit of over-enthusiasm that might endanger the safety of other crewmembers. For example, being stuck in the mud in calm waters might induce some carefree frolicking, with the crew trying their own schemes to free the boat, such as jumping overboard to push while someone else is gunning the engine in forward and reverse gears. Not only can the grounding then become more complicated, but crew safety may be placed in serious question. There is a strong tendency for crewmembers to consider a grounding an excuse for a swimming party, when they will be in the water unprotected. The knowledgeable skipper, realizing that injuries (such as cut feet) will just further complicate an already unfavorable situation, should insist on proper personal protection gear and proper procedures for all crewmembers.

Perhaps more serious are the anxieties that are quite naturally present during a grounding, especially if it was a hard one with complications (e.g., surf moving the boat, the boat taking on water, heeled sharply over). The skipper will want to try to assure the crew and passengers that they will be safe if they follow instructions explicitly.

The skipper must keep attention directed toward the problem in a coordinated way. The best way to do this is to make use of a well-tuned plan for ungrounding. An ungrounding plan should include communications procedures, contingency considerations for abandoning the ungrounding efforts in case of unexpected developments, procedures for recovering anchors and other salvage gear, procedures for relocating once the boat is afloat, and steps to be executed in separate crew tasks.

Individual Tasks and Teamwork

If you have inexperienced passengers aboard, it is best to keep them seated in the cockpit or on the cabin roof until they are asked to do something. A calm, but firm, attitude by the skipper will help to lend credibility to the plan of action. This is not the time to enter into lengthy discussions with passengers on why the boat is disabled, nor is it the time to formulate a joint plan. Of course, passenger suggestions need not be ignored completely, but timing may be critical to avoid compounding the grounding problem. Try to give inexperienced passengers a simple assignment to keep them occupied, such as posting watches or preparing anchor lines.

The crew may also have been jostled around by the grounding and be disoriented. Since they have less knowledge about the craft than you do as skipper, and perhaps little knowledge of refloating techniques, they probably will be awaiting orders. Individual sailors react differently to emergencies, so it is entirely possible that some crewmembers will prove to be less than useful when they are needed most. Fear can be difficult to manage. Recognize this and devise a strategy that works around and with those who are fearful and/or disoriented. Give everyone something to do, even if you just tell them to stay below to report on hull damage.

You will need to develop a team attitude, even if the team consists of only two people. It is simply a matter of working together toward a common goal—in this case, freeing the boat from the bottom. Give clear directions and then observe carefully that each task is completed. Shouting several confusing or incomplete orders at once will only tend to invite more disorder. Insist that crewmembers work together for safety and coordination; this is no time for individual gallantry. Be calm, be firm, be explicit. Have an ever-vigilant attitude, head off danger, and be aware that anything can go wrong. You already have one problem. Don't create additional ones with an undisciplined crew.

Maintaining Healthy Attitudes

Even if your prognosis of the situation is not particularly good, it is important to keep up morale. In a serious grounding, such as one in which there is danger of losing the boat in the surf, passengers and crew will be looking to you as the skipper for immediate guidance. Tell them of the options you are considering. Reinforce the concept that they are better off working together under survival conditions. Keep spirits optimistic.

The Skipper's Role as Disciplinarian

Finally, if necessary, you should be demanding. The skipper is legally responsible for the reasonable safety of the crew (Safe Boating Act of 1971, as amended). If not properly disciplined, crewmembers will often attempt their own remedies and endanger themselves and others. Moreover, such attempts may be counterproductive to other efforts to refloat the boat. Once safe on land, crewmembers are free to do something else; on board during an emergency, the captain is in command—or should be. You cannot justifiably relinquish your responsibilities. Fatalities and injuries often occur during groundings because of a lack of discipline. No one but you should decide when to abandon the boat. That may not make you popular, but you may save lives and prevent injuries—and probably save the boat.

Coast Guard records show an inordinate number of injuries and deaths associated with groundings. The problem probably is related to crew enthusiasm and inexperience. Sailboats, because of their deep keels, usually are stranded in relatively deep water, which adds to the safety problem. Many of the standard refloating techniques are potentially dangerous, so it is essential to exercise care in instructing crewmembers, or others who come to assist, in proper safety procedures. (This is particularly true in night groundings.) Appear confident and be effective.

Full Safety Provisions

Personal flotation devices (PFDs/life jackets) should be mandatory unless the water is so shallow that a person can stand easily. Even then, it is desirable to wear a PFD in case an accident should render a person unconscious. Be on the safe side, give the order to break out PFDs

People working in the water, especially in surf, should use life harnesses or lifelines. This is particularly true for anyone working underwater, such as when securing padding to protect the hull. Also, be sure to tether the dinghy with a painter so that it may be hauled in if the boat capsizes. This is no time to lose the dinghy. Keep on hand a throwable lifering, ready to deploy at a moment's notice, with a 50- to 100-foot line attached. Most cruising boats carry one or two of these on the stern rail, but I notice an absence of retrieving lines.

People in the water should be clothed and always wear footgear. It is a good idea to keep on board a half-dozen pairs of cotton work gloves for all kinds of tasks (like hand-hauling anchor chain), and everyone assisting in ungrounding a boat should wear them.

The Dinghy

The most dangerous part of rowing out a heavy kedge in a dinghy is wrestling with the anchor. Lash it just below the transom with a light line belayed inside the dinghy. Once over the drop zone, simply cut the light line and let it fall. I have bolted two eyes on the transom of our dinghy for this purpose. Setting a kedge from a dinghy is a one-person job; two people and the kedge will jeopardize the stability of the dinghy. Make sure the bitter end of the kedge line is secured to the grounded boat. Coil the line in the dinghy so it can be payed out as the dinghy is rowed, or have a person on deck pay out the line as the kedge is rowed out.

Contacting the Coast Guard

Advise the Coast Guard of your predicament, even if you feel they cannot be of assistance. This way, they will be alerted to your situation if the crew becomes endangered or injured, and they probably will be receiving land-based telephone calls and radio messages regarding your plight. Advise them when you are safely refloated. Ask for assistance if there is any question regarding the safety of the crew. In particularly hazardous situations, they will know what to do and likely will have the necessary equipment to rescue boat and crew. Do not, however, summon a Coast Guard vessel and keep it standing by if you are simply inconvenienced and waiting for the tide to take you off.

The Decision to Abandon

Some, even many, groundings leave no hope for salvaging the boat. In such cases, it is essential to make a timely decision to abandon the boat. Recognize that there are some situations you cannot control, such as being piled up on a rocky lee shore in hurricane-force winds with the boat starting to break up. No matter how reluctant you feel, the best course of action is to save the crew and not worry about the boat.

Much is written about boats abandoned prematurely at sea before every effort was made to save them. This is not the same situation as in a serious grounding during adverse weather conditions, when you have extremely limited control. Obviously, if the potential for loss of life or injury to the crew is not present, then you will endeavor to make every effort to save the boat. But it is senseless to jeopardize or injure a skipper or his crew when desperate conditions prevail.

When your boat goes aground, consider removing to shore as many crewmembers as possible. This is for safety reasons as well as to lighten the boat. And they can also help by securing aid ashore, running lines ashore (when drying out, for example), and doing other work associated with the ungrounding effort. If the boat is to dry out, she will be heeled at such an angle that the crew probably will wish to be ashore anyway. If the grounded boat is not equipped with a dinghy or inflatable, or has somehow lost the use of its tender, try to engage assistance from land or from other boats operating in the vicinity. Swimming ashore, while wearing a PFD, is the last choice. If that is the only option, it would help to float a safety line through the surf on a fender or other buoyed object, to be secured both on the boat and ashore.

Close the Bar

In 1982 there were 1,178 deaths on the American waterways, making boating the second most dangerous mode of travel (after automobiles). The record shows that well over half of these deaths involved the use of alcohol. Make it a rigid rule that the bar is closed during a grounding, and that all partially consumed drinks are discarded. Everyone needs to think clearly during the course of the ungrounding efforts. That also includes crew put ashore, as they may be needed later.

CHAPTER 3

Principles of Buoyancy

Many groundings require only a nominal amount of reduced draft to free the boat. The calculations necessary to determine the value of reducing the gross weight to make a particular boat more buoyant, thus decreasing the distance from the boat's keel to her waterline, are fairly straightforward to prepare, but they are hopelessly time-consuming during most emergency groundings. It pays, then, as was said in Chapter 1, to know the particulars about your boat in advance, and to work out a sound lightening strategy before the keel ever hits the ground.

It was Archimedes, musing in his bathtub one day in 250 B.C., who hit upon the principle of buoyancy: A body partially or completely immersed in a fluid is buoyed up, or sustained, by a force equal to the weight of the fluid displaced. Cork and wood float because they are less dense than the water. Metal, however, is denser. A one-pound chunk of bronze dropped into a tub of water will plummet to the bottom, but if this same pound of bronze is hammered into a thin, shallow bowl, it will float. In the form of a bowl, it is presenting a considerably larger surface to the water, displacing a pound of liquid, and a force equal to the weight of the displaced water is buoying up the bowl.

Every modern ship has a displacement curve plotted by her architects from the lines and hull dimensions. This graph is turned over to

15

her officers on delivery. To gauge the ship's weight or displacement at any time during loading or unloading, they simply take the average of the bow and stern drafts—the vertical distances between the water and the keel. (These measurements are obtained from draft marks spaced every six inches on the bow and stern.) A glance at the graph tells the deck officer the number of tons of water she is displacing. That figure is, of course, the precise equivalent of her own weight plus everything aboard. Conversely, the officers can learn from the graph what her draft will be under any given load.

Effects of Lightening a Boat

Yachts usually do not have the graphs or hull markings of ships, relying instead on hull waterline markings or stripes. The normal loads for small pleasure craft are determined by the designer. Herein lies the problem of calculating the precise level of the keel when displacement is changed by the removal of weight. Each boat has a known displacement, of course, and to this is added the weight of people, fuel, water, equipment, and so forth. The effect on buoyancy—and thus on decreasing the draft of the boat—of removing fluids, people, or other items is dependent on the weight of each thing removed in addition to the buoyancy factor of the craft itself. Thus, each boat must be evaluated individually. Obviously, these kinds of calculations are not normally kept aboard. As a grounded cruising-boat skipper, you would be better advised to use your own rule-of-thumb based on past loading experiences with the boat. The skipper of an unfamiliar boat, such as one borrowed or chartered, is at a distinct disadvantage in this respect.

Very heavily laden live-aboard cruising boats can be down as much as four inches below their designed waterline. It is not uncommon for an owner of such a boat to move the waterline markings to reflect more accurately the boat's normal operating displacement level. The crews of regular racing and cruising boats frequently observe waterline levels under different loads, so they already have a rough idea of where the boat normally sits when she is at her dock or mooring and when she is fully loaded. Boat designers have suggested that a working differential of about two inches of freeboard might be gained by fully unloading a 30-foot sloop, but they are quick to add qualifying factors, such as the density of the mass of the boat.

Nevertheless, if the boat is in a grounding situation where a small difference in draft might assist in freeing her, then by all means consider lightening the boat. This could be especially useful on a rocky or coral bottom where only a small part of the keel could be wedged tightly. Then, too, a lighter boat is easier to tow, kedge, or heel.

A normal cruising boat should be able to remove quite easily more than 1,000 pounds of people, water, spare ground tackle (including all chain), heavy tools, extra sails, and other extra gear. Water tank lines can be uncoupled to allow the water to flow to the bilge, from where it can be pumped overboard (8.3 pounds per gallon). In a serious emergency, most of the fuel can be jettisoned. (Frequently a pump hose may be inserted in an inspection port on top of the tank.)

Adding External Buoyancy

It is also possible to add external buoyancy to a grounded boat. This is rarely done, but it can be another tool at your disposal, especially in complicated situations. Commercial salvors often use buoyancy containers or air bags in many different salvage operations, including raising sunken ships. Most such buoyancy devices are cumbersome for small boats to carry, although emergency inflatable rubber bags are available on the pleasure-boat market.

Coast Guard rescue boats carry emergency flotation bags to use as external buoyancy to keep small boats from sinking. These 60-by-38-inch bags, resembling a pillow when inflated, provide 500 pounds of buoyancy. They are inflated with cans of liquid freon, which, when activated, changes to a gas.

The U.S. Navy has larger inflatable salvage pontoons. The pontoon provides buoyancy for lifting submerged objects and may be used separately or in a series of three. The inflated dimensions are 86 inches in diameter and 121 inches in length (folding size is 70 by 54 by 20 inches), providing 8.4 long tons of buoyancy. The dry weight of 750 pounds makes them cumbersome for use with a small boat. U.S. Navy salvage units occasionally participate in yacht ungroundings as part of their training or to assist other authorities in clearing navigable waterways. There are naval salvage training facilities in Virginia, Florida, and California, as well as a number of Mobile Diving and Salvage Units (MDSU) at U.S. Navy bases around the country.

The rigging required to hold flotation devices in place below the waterline is extensive and normally beyond the capability of most small-boat crews. It is conceivable, however, that when all else fails, especially in remote locations where commercial assistance might be unavailable, it might be worth the effort to add external buoyancy in an attempt to refloat a boat.

In the absence of the containers made for this purpose, innovative techniques and devices must be used. It may be necessary to rig slings under the hull and attach barrels, heavy timbers, or whatever else is around. Large construction companies sometimes own inflatable pontoon platforms, and diving firms often have suitable air compressors. In one grounding case, more than 200 heavy-duty garbage bags inflated and placed under the hull added the buoyancy needed to lift a large wooden sailboat. The potential solutions are limited only by your own imagination.

CHAPTER 4

Using the Tides

The local tidal range and its existing stage are of principal interest to the skipper and/or salvager of any vessel grounded in tidal waters, so it is essential to know your tides. A boat grounded on an ebb tide may have to wait a full 12-hour tide cycle before it can be floated again. In such cases, the decreasing water level brings the potential of additional damage to the boat. If the boat is aground on a flood tide, then the problem is different, but not necessarily easier. Wave and wind action often drive the vessel farther ashore into an even more difficult position.

But things could be worse. You could be beneaped, the condition of a vessel left aground by a spring tide, too high for the following neap tide to refloat her. Since the spring tide is the highest high water, a vessel so grounded may very well have to wait for the next spring tide. Spring tides occur twice monthly, with the new moon and the full moon, on the Atlantic coast of the United States. There have been cases where boats stranded at high springs in remote locations of the world had to be abandoned forever because of this phenomenon.

On an ebbing tide, quick action is required before the boat is hopelessly aground. In an area with a tidal range of 12 feet, for example, you can often expect a fall of 4 inches in 10 minutes. In almost all cases, if the tide level is less than what was present when you went aground, you should prepare to wait until that level is reached again.

The Tidal Phenomenon

Although we have all learned about tides and their effects at one time or another, they are so crucial to the subject of going aground that it is worth reviewing the basics of the tidal phenomenon.

Tides are caused by the differences in attractive forces of various celestial bodies, essentially the moon and the sun, upon different parts of the rotating earth. To the mariner these periodic motions of the oceans of the world can be an aid or a hindrance. They may help him clear a bar at a harbor entrance, for example, or prevent him from entering a harbor. Similarly, the tidal currents that accompany the rise and fall of the tides may help his progress through the water or hinder it; they may set him toward or away from dangers. Tide is the vertical rise and fall of the water, while current is the horizontal flow. The relationship between these is not simple, nor is it the same everywhere in the world.

To understand what causes tides, consider the earth and the moon. The moon appears to revolve about the earth, but actually the moon and earth revolve about their common center of mass. They are held together by gravitational attraction and kept apart by an equal and opposite centrifugal force. In this earth-moon system, the tide-producing force on the earth's hemisphere that is nearer the moon is in the direction of the moon's attraction, or toward the moon. On the hemisphere that is farther from the moon, the tide-producing force is in the direction of the centrifugal force, or away from the moon. The tide-producing forces, then, tend to create high tides on the sides of the earth nearest to and farthest from the moon, with a low-tide belt between them. Changes in the declination of the moon create inequality of the tidal forces at a particular place. Similar forces are produced by the sun, and the total tide-producing force is a result of the two. Sizes and shapes of ocean basins and the interference of land masses prevent the tides from assuming a simple, regular pattern.

The maximum-height high tide and the minimum-level low tide are properly referred to as high water and low water. A semidiurnal type of tide is formed on the Atlantic coast of the United States. This type of tide has two highs and two lows each tidal day, with the highs and the lows being nearly equal. A diurnal type of tide, which has a single high and a single low each tidal day, occurs in such locales as the north shore of the Gulf of Mexico. And, finally, there is a mixed type of tide, combining the above, which usually has two high and two low waters each tidal day, but occasionally the tide may become diurnal or have great inequalities in heights of the two highs or the two lows. These mixed tides are prevalent along the Pacific coast of the United States.

Although the tide at a particular place can be classified by type, it exhibits many variations during the month. The range of the tide varies in accordance with the intensity of the tide-producing force, although there may be a lag of a day or two (age of tide) between a particular astronomic cause and its tidal effect. Thus, when the moon is at the point in its orbit nearest the earth (at perigee), the lunar semi-diurnal range is increased, and perigean tides occur. This greater tidal range can be of benefit in freeing a grounded boat. When the moon is farthest from the earth (at apogee), smaller apogean tides occur. When the moon and sun are in line and pulling together, as at new moon and full moon, spring tides occur. (The term *spring* in this context has nothing to do with the season of the year, derived from the ancient verb *springen*—to leap up.) When the moon and the sun oppose each other, as at the quadratures (90-degree angles from the sun), the smaller neap tides occur. When certain of these phenomena coincide, the great perigean spring tides, the small apogean neap tides, and other irregularities occur.

Tidal Datums

A tidal datum is a level from which heights and depths are measured. The National Ocean Survey (NOS) tide tables show the relation of the tide each day during a month to these datums for certain places. The most important level of reference to sailors is the datum of soundings on charts. These show depths below a selected low-water datum. Tide predictions in tide tables show heights above that same level. To determine the depth of water available at a specific time, you just add the height of the tide at the time in question to the charted depth (or subtract the predicted height if the charted figure is negative).

By international agreement, the level used as a chart datum should be just low enough so that low waters do not go far below it. At many places, however, the level used is one determined from a mean of a number of low waters (usually over a 19-year period), so some low waters can be expected to be even lower. Below are some of the datums in general use.

The highest low-water datum in general use, including the United States, is mean low water (MLW), which is the average height of all low waters at one place, with about half the low waters falling below it. Mean low water springs (MLWS), usually referred to as low water springs, is the average level of the low waters that occur at the times of spring tides. Mean lower low water (MLLW) is the average height of the lower low waters at a location. Tropic lower low water (TLLW) is the average height of lower low waters that occur when the moon is near maximum declination and the diurnal effect is most pronounced. Lowest normal low water is a datum that approximates the average height of monthly lowest low waters. In some areas of the world where there is little or no tide, mean sea level is used as chart datum, being the average height of the surface of the sea for all stages of the tide over a 19-year period.

One reason many boats go aground is a misunderstanding of the charted depths. The charted depths may vary by several feet or more from the actual water depths at a place because of the way the datum is averaged. Moreover, the meteorological effects of other than normal weather can change predicted tidal levels considerably. The level of the sea is affected by wind and atmospheric pressure. As a general rule, onshore winds raise the sea level and offshore winds lower it, but the amount of change varies at different places. During periods of low atmospheric pressure, the water tends to be higher than normal. Where a tidal range is very small, the meteorological effect may sometimes be greater than the normal tide. In Eastport, Maine, for example, the effects of weather can easily produce three or four additional feet of water. And since Eastport's 30-foot tidal range is the greatest in the United States, averaging means that there might be three or four feet less water at certain low tides. Obviously, this is significant when you consider that a grounded boat may need only a couple of additional inches of water to break free.

Tide Tables

Tide tables for various parts of the world are published in four volumes by the U.S. Coast and Geodetic Survey. A complete explanation of how to use the tables is contained in each volume. Each volume is arranged as follows:

Table 1 contains a complete list of the predicted times and heights of the tide for each day of the year at a number of places designated as reference stations.

Table 2 gives differences and ratios that can be used to modify the tidal information for the reference stations to make it applicable to a relatively large number of subordinate stations.

Table 3 provides information for use in finding the approximate height of the tide at any time between high and low water.

Table 4 is a sunrise-sunset table at five-day intervals for various latitudes.

Table 5 provides an adjustment to convert the local mean time of Table 4 to zone or standard time.

Table 6 gives the zone time of moonrise and moonset for each day of the year at selected places.

Table 7 gives certain astronomical data.

The principal use of the Tide Tables is to keep boats from going aground. If you are sailing in oceans or tidal backwaters, it is necessary to use the Tide Tables for predicting tide levels because of the many calculations involved. The principal use of the Tide Tables for boats already aground is to determine when there will be enough water to refloat the boat. This can be a critical calculation if the boat has gone aground at high tide, especially a spring high tide.

The Rule of Twelfths

A handy, but less accurate, way to estimate the height of the tide at any time is by using the Rule of Twelfths. If the tidal range is 8 feet, for example, and the time between tides is 6 hours, the amount of change during the first hour will be $\frac{1}{12}$ (or 8 percent) of 8 feet—or 8 inches. During the second hour the change will be $\frac{2}{12}$ (17 percent) of 8 feet—or 1 foot 4 inches. The total accumulated hourly change during this interval will, of course, equal the total range. Thus:

1st sixth of range	1/12	(8%)
2nd sixth of range	2/12	(17%)
3rd sixth of range	3/12	(25%)
4th sixth of range	3/12	(25%)
5th sixth of range	2/12	(17%)
6th sixth of range	1/12	(8%)

Aground on a Spring Tide

If the boat is beneaped, i.e., grounded at a spring high tide, it may be necessary to wait two weeks or more for the new or full moon before she can be refloated, depending on the tidal range. In that case, it is worth trying to find another solution. For example, it may be possible to lift the boat off with a crane that is onshore or on a barge. If the situation is serious enough, it may even be possible to dig a trench in the bottom with a backhoe to refloat her, probably with some extra nudging. To do this, it will be necessary to make careful calculations, taking into consideration the age of tide, as mentioned above. Remember that less than an inch of clearance under the keel can free your boat.

In July 1903, a large sailboat went aground in Boston Harbor. The amazed crew, thinking they were off course, abandoned the boat. The sailboat was already afloat by the time the Coast Guard vessel got to the scene one-half hour later; aboard they found $2 million worth of marijuana. It was a spring low and the boat was in the right place but in the wrong hands.

Tidal Currents

The daily rise and fall of the tide, with its attendant flood and ebb of tidal current, is familiar to every sailor. He is also aware that at high water and low water the depth of the water is momentarily constant, a condition called *stand.* Similarly, there is a moment of slack water as the tidal current reverses direction. As a general rule, the change in height or current speed is at first very slow, increasing to a maximum about midway between the two tidal extremes. If plotted against time, the height of tide or speed of a tidal current takes the general form of a sine curve.

When your boat is grounded, tidal currents usually do not work to your advantage. If you are caught aground in a narrow channel in a fast-moving tidal current, perhaps enhanced by the outflow of a river, the current will tend to turn the relatively wide and deep keel of a sailboat broadside to the current, sometimes burying the lee toerail in the swiftly moving water. Thus, the boat simply pivots on the point of grounding. If you are on the outer bend of the channel, the current will try to drive your boat farther aground. Currents that follow shorelines may tend to keep a grounded boat from freeing herself.

In some places, tidal currents reach 8 or 9 knots. It is a serious problem to tow or kedge off a grounded boat during the high-velocity period, so if possible, it is better to wait until the high stand or slack-water period. A grounded boat ungrounded in such strong currents can easily get out of control and immediately go aground again, perhaps with more serious consequences. Currents, both tidal and nontidal, are also important considerations in refloating by kedging or towing. More about this appears in Chapter 10.

CHAPTER 5

Lights and Signals

According to the international-inland Rules of the Road, boats aground shall exhibit an all-round white light where it can best be seen, in addition to two all-round red lights in a vertical line and three black balls in a vertical line (Rule 30, Rules of the Road, International-Inland). However, the rule waives these requirements for vessels of less than 12 meters (39.37 feet) in length when aground in locations other than in or near a narrow channel, fairway, or anchorage, or where other vessels normally navigate. This is a newer provision that recognizes that smaller vessels have difficulty carrying the lights and shapes specified.

A Homebuilt Signal Light

No one seems to deny the need for one required all-round white light at night if grounded, and this can be accomplished quite easily by hanging an anchor light where it can be seen best. Few boats tend to be equipped to meet the provision of two all-round red lights in a vertical line. This is unfortunate, because the operator of a larger vessel, for instance, in adhering to the strict application of the rules, would have no way of assessing the situation of a grounded boat not displaying the two red lights.

To comply with this provision, I have rigged two red 360-degree lenses between three round pieces of wood and installed common

12-volt car bulb sockets. The whole thing is held together with a long, threaded ⁵⁄₁₆-inch shaft (available in all hardware stores). Small drilled holes at both ends of the bolt hold stainless rings. A long electric cord is designed to allow the lamp to be hoisted to spreader height, port or starboard.

Signaling Other Vessels

The prudent mariner will keep in mind Rule 36, Signals to Attract Attention, when aground at night. Any vessel may make light or sound signals, ones that cannot be mistaken for any authorized signal, to attract attention. If you focus a searchlight in the direction of an approaching ship, for instance, that will help assure that your situation is noticed before you are run down. Obviously, *you* cannot move.

The three-black-ball requirement for a grounded vessel can be satisfied in a number of ways, but since these are not readily available commercially in the United States, I simply use three round aluminum radar reflectors painted black. They fold flat when not in use. Once again, this is a signal that other vessels will be looking for if you are in a regularly used waterway.

The Boat's Bell

The boat's bell is used once every minute to give the aground sound signal. The pattern is three separate and distinct strokes of the bell, followed by the rapid ringing of the bell, and then immediately followed by three additional strokes of the bell. (Repeated short whistle blasts may also be sounded to avoid collisions.) Vessels of less than 40 feet in length are not required to give this signal, but if they do not, they must make some other efficient sound signal not more than every two minutes. Rule 36, Signals to Attract Attention, is also useful here. Any sound signal, like blasts from an airhorn, should be used to avoid a collision. It may be that approaching vessels do not know that you are aground and will be following the Rules of the Road, conceivably creating a dangerous situation. Do whatever it takes to avoid a collision, a crisis that would further complicate an already unfavorable situation.

Flags

The art of signaling by international flags and pennants is not dead, although it is used infrequently in these days of good VHF radio communications. The flag display, always flown where it can be seen most easily by the receiving station, is most valuable to ships, which always carry a copy of the *International Code of Signals* (DMA Publication number 102) on the bridge. The flag signals on groundings are quite extensive, having been developed since 1857, when the first *International Code* was published. Some of the signals for groundings, for instance, are to alert another vessel that she is in danger of going aground. For the small-boat operator, the flags "JG" (I am aground; I am in a dangerous situation) or "JH" (I am aground; I am not in danger) should suffice. (See Appendix D for a complete listing of signals used in grounding situations.)

PART TWO

BASIC TECHNIQUES

CHAPTER 6

Hard Aground

The reasons why you are aground are unimportant right now. Later you can analyze the circumstances and conditions that helped cause the incident. You will soon know what did it, such as a miscalculated tide level, stronger-than-expected currents that set you toward low depths, a strong gust that put you off course, or just inaccurate piloting. The important thing is that you know what actions should be taken immediately.

The types of groundings cover a wide range, of course, from those where the yacht immediately starts to break up on a rocky lee shore to the common stuck-in-the-mud type. Because each grounding is unique, a great deal rests on the skipper's judgment. The ungrounding or salvage techniques that best apply to a given situation must be evaluated and applied in a timely fashion to be successful. A great deal of ingenuity and resourcefulness may be in order, given the limited amount of heavy lines and other gear a small boat is able to carry for such emergencies.

If you are unfortunate enough to be stranded, you should use whatever ungrounding techniques you deem appropriate, alone or in combination. Study the situation carefully, make an operations plan, and note exactly where the keel is aground and where you would like to be when ungrounded. The keel may be touching at only one small point, for example, where pivoting the boat may free it. The place where you want to go should be such that you can successfully execute a workable plan. Be persistent. In almost all cases there is a way to save the boat or at least mitigate damage so the boat may be salvaged later. Do not relax your vigil until you are safely on your way again, assured that there is no significant damage. Many a minor grounding has turned into a disaster because of changes in weather or waves, slow initial responses, lack of safety precautions, and other forces beyond the control of the crew, such as ship wakes and unexpected strong currents. No matter how minor, do not underestimate the seriousness of any grounding.

Using the Engine

The immediate reaction of almost all pleasure-boat skippers upon grounding is to reverse the engine to pull the boat off. (See Figure 3.) This sometimes works well if it is a simple grounding in soft mud or sand under tranquil conditions. But the relatively heavy weight of moving sailboats or heavy powerboats usually puts their keels so hard aground that the engine alone will not do the trick. Fixed sailboat

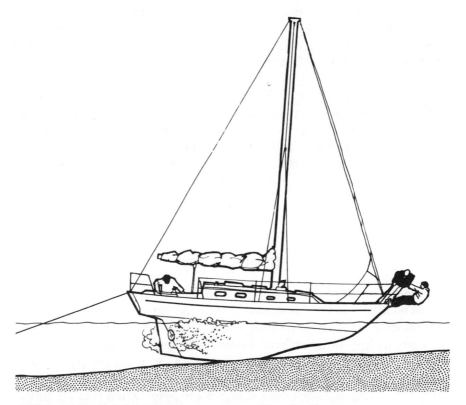

Figure 3. Backing off under power, with a kedge set and weight shifted, sometimes will free a stranded boat.

propellers in reverse gear attain only 60 percent of their forward thrust, folding or low-drag propellers even less. Using the engine can stir up bottom material, which can quickly clog engine water intake valves and hoses. Powerboat propellers and engine water intakes usually are even less protected. Keep a sharp eye on the engine water temperature gauge during all use of the engine to detect a clogging situation. To clean the intake, close the seacock, unclamp the hose at the seacock and the water pump, and blow or force wire through the hose to dislodge debris. A swimmer can clean the port entrance with a short length of wire. The water pump itself may have to be disassembled to be cleaned. The indiscriminate hard use of the engine while trying to extricate your grounded boat may seriously damage the powerplant.

Controlling Pounding

The possibility of damage beyond the initial impact is present in all groundings. Pounding and broaching are two ever-present dangers. Pounding is caused by varying the degree of buoyancy of a grounded boat. The waterline changes constantly with succeeding crests and troughs of waves, thus producing an alternating increase and decrease in the boat's total buoyancy. When this condition is great enough to lift the boat off the bottom and drop it back again, hull damage can occur. Such damage may range from a few open seams to the serious holing of the grounded boat. Each wave striking against the boat tends to drive it farther aground. However, the alert skipper can take advantage of this momentary ungrounding to free the boat by kedging or motoring, or by being towed off.

Broaching

Broaching, caused by surf hitting a boat on the side or quarter, results in the boat being thrown broadside. This is particularly dangerous for two reasons: (1) broaching tends to drive the boat harder aground, and (2) currents are set up around the bow and the stern of the boat. The velocity of these currents will scour sand away from the boat's hull, piling it up to leeward amidships, thus leaving the boat supported only amidships. This is sometimes called a *tombolo*. When this condition exists, the keel of the boat often breaks, rendering the boat a total loss. Attempts to refloat should be avoided in this case.

The Importance of Preparation

As mentioned briefly in Chapter 1, if you are a prepared skipper, you will have a plan of action even before going aground. You should be able to accept a grounding as one of the inevitable hazards associated with boating, so you should be able to resolve the problem with the same confident spirit you have shown in many other sailing endeavors. Of course you will be disappointed in your seamanship for allowing the incident to happen, even if it is beyond your control, but there should be no discernible confusion or fear. Self-confidence will prevail if the unexpected is anticipated. It is all part of good seamanship.

Hazards to an Aiding Boat

It is not uncommon to see a grounded boat and want to offer help. It is also possible to see two grounded boats you may want to help, the second one being a would-be salvor. Avoid the obvious problem of going aground yourself, as it will just complicate everyone's day. There are steps that can be taken, however, to assist a grounded boat while standing off in deeper water. Giving advice is one possible aid, if the skipper of the disabled boat has little knowledge of refloating techniques. (But do not be disappointed if all your suggestions are not heeded.) If weather conditions are appropriate, you might anchor off and wait for a request for assistance. Boats moving back and forth near a stranded vessel are of no assistance; in fact, they are often a distracting factor. It would be considerate to take your dinghy over to the grounded boat to offer assistance. It may be, for example, that they may not have a dinghy available to take soundings or row out a kedge, or extra ground tackle might be welcomed. Naturally, you do not want to employ any ungrounding techniques without the skipper's approval.

Even a low-powered auxiliary sailboat may be useful in towing a grounded boat off the bottom, especially if the assisting boat has set an anchor in the direction of the pull to gain additional power, in conjunction with other efforts by the disabled boat. Follow all towing safety precautions, described in Chapter 10. Know the limitations of your towing gear and deck hardware. Know when to abort a tow because the disabled boat is too firmly aground, an ebbing tide has reduced water levels, or the available gear cannot safely take the strain of the tow.

Be prepared to assist in removing crew and gear from the grounded boat if requested. The original grounding conditions can deteriorate quickly with adverse weather conditions, a building surf, a holed hull, and so forth. Consider stringing a sturdy line between the two vessels to assist with crew abandonment. Also, the grounded boat may wish to remove gear to gain buoyancy. The skippers must, however, be alert to the inherent dangers to crew safety when the two boats are in close proximity, such as crewmembers attempting to leap from one deck to the other or fending off with feet or hands.

In some cases, the bulk weight of the aiding boat's crewmembers might be used to shift the keel of the grounded boat. Or that same crew might offer to go overboard and push. A properly anchored aiding boat might well be able to assist in a careening maneuver by running a masthead line from the stranded boat through its most powerful winch. This, of course, depends on the ability of the aiding boat to be located in a proper position without being endangered.

Then, too, just the beneficial psychological effects of knowing help is nearby can often boost crew morale on the grounded boat and lessen the anxiety, thus allowing maneuvers to proceed efficiently.

Underwater Survey

If conditions are suitable and a diver or underwater swimmer is available, it is a good idea to inspect the hull, keel, and rudder for damage and to attempt to determine the points where the boat is grounded. It is also desirable to inspect the bottom for rocks, ledges, or other obstructions that might hamper pulling the boat off or might damage the hull should she be dried out.

CHAPTER 7

Kedging Off

Kedging off, the process of freeing the boat with an anchor, called a kedge, is as old as recorded history. Usually, the easiest and best way off is the same route the boat went aground. Your regular service anchor will do as a kedge if you are not driven too hard on the bottom; otherwise, the heaviest anchor you have, or can borrow, should be set firmly in the direction of deep water.

It is best to set the anchor a considerable distance away from the grounded boat to ensure that the best possible scope is obtained. This way, the kedge is more apt to dig deeply into the bottom and will take advantage of a reduced angle between the belaying point on the craft and the bottom, thus increasing horizontal pull (as opposed to a shorter scope, which tends to pull the boat's bow section down). Longer scope also allows more maneuvering room once the boat breaks free.

Rowing or Swimming Out the Kedge

First, take soundings in the direction of deep water, as described in Chapter 1, to determine the best location for the kedge. Use of unverified information can result in much wasted time and effort.

The kedge can be rowed out in a dinghy or any other small boat. (See Figure 4.) Frequently, small boats come to the aid of a grounded boat, so it may be possible to have another party set the kedge while rode is payed out from the grounded vessel. If a dinghy is used, it is best to load the anchor and a substantial portion of the anchor line

35

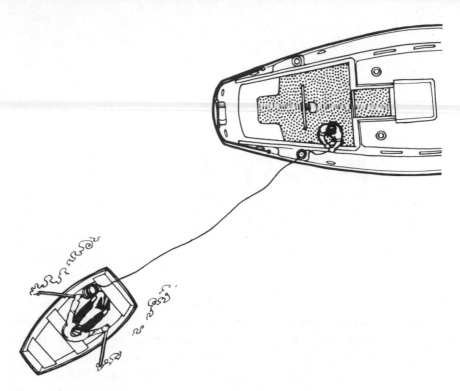

Figure 4. It usually is best to set a kedge anchor by rowing it out in a dinghy, feeding the line from the dinghy.

aboard before rowing out, as towing the line through the water is cumbersome and could upset the dinghy. The best way to handle the anchor is to lash it to the dinghy transom with light line, which you then cut to drop the anchor once you are over the desired location. Have one or more through-bolted cleats or rings in your dinghy that can be used to secure the kedge line. This task should be performed by a single person to maintain maximum stability of the dinghy. It is not uncommon for a dinghy to capsize while carrying a kedge, so the operator should be wearing a life jacket.

In an emergency, in the absence of a small boat, a kedge can be lashed to anything that will support it in the water: logs, planks, several life preservers tied together, and so forth. A swimmer (wearing shoes) can then push the kedge out to a desired location while another person pays out the anchor line. A second swimmer can assist in towing the line, which can have considerable resistance in the water. If no one is available to assist, the line should be coiled on the deck so that it can be dragged free more easily.

A Winch for the Kedge

Once the kedge is set, it should be rove through a chock and led to the boat's most powerful winch, with blocks to reduce friction if necessary. Here is where some innovative rigging may be in order. If the boat went aground bow first and the deepest water lies to port astern, for example, then the kedge line should exert pulling power in that direction. If the boat is equipped with a powerful anchor winch, then the line should be run forward. Modern sheet winches often have tremendous pulling power. A handybilly can be rigged if large winches are not available. Many seasoned skippers carry aboard a come-along, a portable winch sold in most hardware and automotive stores. More than one kedge can be set for added pulling power.

Setting the Kedge(s) Quickly

It is important in most groundings that the kedge be set immediately. This increases the chances of freeing the craft before the keel works its way deeper into the bottom, or before an ebb tide puts the boat hard aground, and it also helps keep the boat from being driven farther ashore by wind, surf, and currents. In many simple groundings, kedging—perhaps combined with propeller thrust—will free a grounded

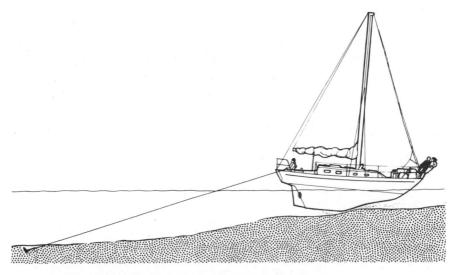

Figure 5. Sometimes it is possible to free a boat just by shifting weight and using a light kedge.

boat. The kedge will also help the operator to maintain some control over the vessel once she is freed. A crewmember should be stationed at the kedge line to take in slack and avoid fouling the propeller once the craft has broken free. Remember that the thrust of a fixed propeller running in reverse will only have about 60 percent of its forward thrust, and there is less if the propeller is a low-drag or folding propeller. Moving the rudder from side to side may also help wiggle the boat and break the keel free from the bottom. It also helps to redistribute weight —crewmembers, gear, whatever is movable. (See Figure 5.)

Waves from a passing boat or ship may lift a grounded boat sufficiently to allow her to be pulled or motored free. Where the grounding is a simple one, such as being lightly aground with the boat showing pivoting movement, it is often possible to have a powerboat make a few close passes to create waves. As the grounded boat lifts and falls with the resultant waves, the keel sometimes is lifted clear of the bottom, allowing the boat to be kedged or powered off. Normal wave action may produce the same effect. After a few attempts, you will soon know if this technique will work. If not, then do not waste time with this approach, but proceed with another ungrounding technique.

CHAPTER 8

Shifting the Keel

Refloating your boat often is a matter of shifting the keel from its grounded position, and several techniques can be used to reach the goal. By heeling the boat to one side, for example, the draft can be reduced just enough to free the keel from the bottom. A substantial tilting is usually necessary, however, because the draft is greatest when the boat is stopped. Also, the keel was probably forced into the bottom either by the weight of the boat if grounded while moored or by forward ramming motion if the boat was underway. If the boat was under sail when it went aground, the keel already was tilted to one side, thereby drawing less water.

It is important to be prepared to move a grounded boat into deeper water once the keel is free from the bottom, since a sailboat refloated by heeling can be driven farther ashore by currents or wind, or simply by drifting. (See Figure 6.) The trick is to know in advance exactly where you want to move the boat, making sure through soundings that you will not run aground again, then working expeditiously to unground her. Be sure to consider the forces of currents and wind working with or against your plan. Also know what you will do once you are in water of adequate floating depth, i.e., anchor, power away, drift with the current. Plan ahead.

Move the boat from side to side to try to determine where the keel is grounded. (The usual grounding while underway often puts just the forward point aground.) This will help you to determine the best direction to heel the boat. Shift people and heavy movable gear all the way forward or aft, depending on the grounding point.

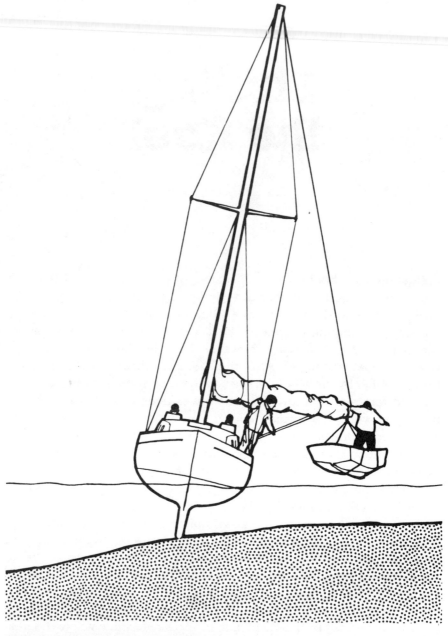

Figure 6. Weight placed on the end of the boom will help in heeling efforts.

Sallying

If she still will not budge despite strain on the kedge and/or engine, try sallying. Place all the movable weight on the port or starboard side and then move it very quickly all at once to the opposite side. This alone sometimes will free a boat from a simple grounding.

In the days of sailing ships, sallying was a common technique for extricating the keel from a muddy or sandy bottom. The crew would be assembled on one side and, on command, would race to the opposite side as the kedge was drawn taut. A few rounds of this and the ship would come free from the suction of the bottom. Navies the world over still place personnel where their body weight will contribute best to freeing the keel in a grounding situation. It is another tried-and-proven technique in your bag of tricks.

Weight on the End of the Boom

Another common technique for heeling a grounded sailboat is to place weight on a swung-out boom. Usually the weight consists of one or more crewmembers who place themselves on the boom while it is amidships, then swing out perpendicular to the boat, controlling lines kept inboard. Weights may be hoisted to the end of the boom with a sheet block or a block rigged specially for that purpose. An anchor will do for a weight, but the likelihood of success is greater if you partially fill a dinghy with water and tether it by a bridled line rove through a block on the boom end and led to a cockpit sheet winch. Once the line is winched in, a substantial heeling strain should result. This is often sufficient to free the keel.

Heeling with a Masthead Line

A slightly more complicated method is to use a masthead line to heel the boat. A halyard with a swivel block at the masthead can be taken to a halyard winch or a sheet winch. Alternatives are the jib and main halyards, but these usually have fixed masthead blocks, making it difficult, if not impossible, to winch in such lines when under heavy strain from either side of the boat. Moreover, such fixed blocks could be damaged, and if wire cables are used, they can be damaged irreparably by twisting and kinking. If ample line is available, it is possible to hoist a loose bowline to the spreaders with a halyard, taking the bitter

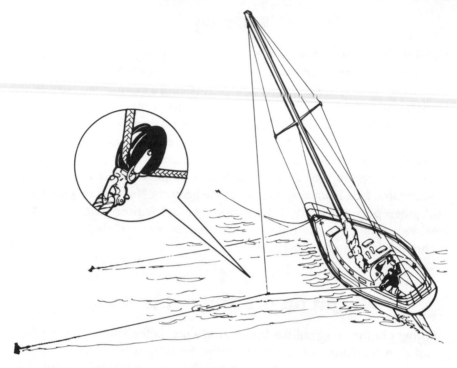

Figure 7. In an attempt to heel a grounded boat,
a deck or mast winch can be used to reel in a halyard
rove through a block attached to an anchor line.

end off the side of the boat to be heeled. The line is rove through a
snatchblock tied to a line from the kedge, then taken to a sheet winch.
(See Figure 7.)

The outboard end of the masthead heeling line should be taken as
far from the side of the boat as possible, with whatever line is available, to provide a better mechanical advantage. It may be taken ashore
if you are close enough and if the pull would be in the right direction.
You can use people in the water to pull on the line, or an adjacent
anchored boat can place strain on the line. Frequently, however, there
is no such handy solution, so the masthead line must be held by an
anchor set for this purpose. The best arrangement for doing this is to
secure the anchor line to a block midway between the boat and the set
anchor. Through this block is rove the masthead line, which is then
taken aboard the grounded boat, preferably to a powerful winch. There
is a very favorable mechanical advantage in heeling by using a pull
from the masthead, but it helps to add to this whatever movable
weight is available on the side of the boat to be heeled.

Heeling the Boat with Sails

Less demanding, but often effective, is the use of sails for heeling a grounded boat after a kedge has been set. If properly done, in sufficiently strong winds from the right direction (usually offshore), this technique can help drive the boat forward and free of the bottom. The sails may be backed, where appropriate, to assist in heeling and moving the vessel, especially in a bow-aground situation. The use of sails, perhaps combined with kedging, towing, people in the water pushing, using the engine, lightening the boat, just might get your boat refloated.

Know crew limitations when using sails during a grounding, especially in delegating this responsibility while you are occupied with some other task. Improper sailhandling in this procedure can drive the boat farther ashore and otherwise complicate an already tricky situation. The normal first step in a grounding on a lee shore with sails set is to furl all sails. The reason for this, of course, is to prevent the sail power from moving the boat about, possibly forcing the boat more firmly aground. But a quick-thinking skipper can use that sail power to take him off the bottom, depending in large measure on his sailhandling skills. In addition, crew can be shifted to the lee rail to aid in the effort. Naturally, this requires that you know your rig well, know how it will behave, and are prepared to demonstrate some extraordinary seamanship. If you have doubts, furl the sails and use other techniques to extricate the boat.

Combining Techniques

Add to the heeling other ungrounding techniques in order to find a combination that may do the job. This heeling technique is well proven and often is all that is needed to refloat a grounded vessel. It will not make up for much of the absolute loss of water from a falling tide, but where the tide range is negligible, it may shorten the waiting time. Heel the boat over hard, with water to the toerail if possible, to break the keel free. (See Figure 8.) If there is still some dragging on the ground, try using people in the water pushing. Secure a tow and/or set a second kedge anchor. Try any or all of the keel-shifting techniques discussed in this chapter and you have a good shot at freeing your boat.

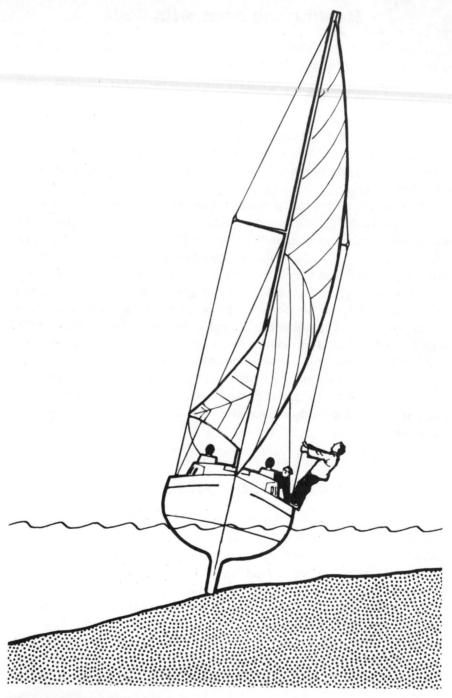

Figure 8. A backed sail can be used to
heel the boat to free the keel.

CHAPTER 9

Controlling Damage

The doctrine of damage control, "hold what you have," also applies to groundings. Prompt efforts to contain progressive flooding, check its source, and shore structural members under added stress can prevent further complications. Moreover, each cubic foot of water (64 pounds) adds weight, which reduces buoyancy and holds the boat more firmly against the bottom. Such added weight exacerbates the grounding and can well make the difference between success and failure in ungrounding attempts.

It is unfortunately true that many grounded boats are lost for lack of simple damage-control action. Few boats, for example, are adequately equipped to deal with hull failure after experiencing a grounding—or, for that matter, during rough weather at sea, collisions, or other unforeseeable problems. Any grounding is complicated by damage that allows water to enter the hull. If the damage is severe enough, under particularly adverse conditions, the boat may have to be abandoned. Fortunately, however, the damage often is less severe than first suspected.

The first action in any grounding is to assess thoroughly the hull damage. If water is flowing in, it must be stopped, and the water already in the hull must be removed. Both measures are important, because the water in the hull affects the boat's stability and also may find its way to the engine and batteries, causing failures that will further complicate the situation. Since there is always the possibility that help will not be available immediately, you should be as self-sufficient as possible. Such an emergency will be less frightening and perhaps less hazardous if some preparation has already been made.

Damage-Control Kit

Every boat should have its own damage-control kit. At the very minimum, carry enough tools and spare parts to make preliminary repairs. Such a kit should include: (1) silicone rubber for plugging holes and seams (it sticks to wet surfaces and will set up under water); (2) Scotch Brand #33 Plastic Tape (it can be applied under water and never slips, unless exposed to oil or gasoline); (3) replacement hoses for every size employed on board and a supply of suitable clamps; (4) soft wooden plugs (unpainted, to absorb water and expand) for every through-hull fitting; (5) canvas, approximately 4 feet by 4 feet; (6) rubber sheet, approximately 4 feet by 4 feet; (7) rags and blankets; (8) tarred marline, at least 200 feet; (9) a mallet; (10) soft wooden wedges or equivalent (shingles), about 15 inches long (unpainted); (11) assorted pieces of lumber, about 3 inches by 3 inches, for shoring; (12) bolt cutter; (13) hand saw.

Patching restores a holed boat's watertight integrity. A good patch is one that resists the foreseen hydrostatic pressure, is located so ambient pressure aids in seating it, and remains in position until permanent repairs are made.

Patching materials and methods are dictated by accessibility, size, and location of the hole. For small holes and cracks, wooden plugs and wedges, oakum, cement, and plastic pastes have been used with success. On moderate-sized holes, groups of plugs and wedges, mattresses, pillows, wood, and metal in combination are common. Large holes require specially designed and carefully constructed patches made from wooden planking or perhaps strong plastic materials, something best executed on a dried-out hull. Poured concrete in prebuilt forms inside the hull makes an effective patch and reinforces external plate patches. Regardless of size, all patches must be mechanically watertight. A cloth or rubber gasket is essential to ensure a watertight seal around the edges of the patch, since the hull surface near a hole may be curved or irregular. Hold patches in place with inside shoring, external ropes and mats, or through-bolts. Butterfly nuts facilitate tightening. In some situations it may be possible to use large screws driven into the hull, although this usually requires predrilling screw holes.

The difficulties in making jury (temporary) repairs to a hull are that patches cannot be nailed to steel or fiberglass hulls, and the curved surfaces on which you are working make the seating of patches difficult. As mentioned above, small holes often can be repaired temporarily by driving in unpainted, soft wooden plugs or wedges. If you wrap the plugs with rags, you will get an additional seal. *Important: Do not drive wedges into cracks, because they will cause the crack to enlarge and expand.* To fill a crack, use silicone rubber and lay a flat piece of rubber and/or canvas over the crack, back it up with a board, and hold the patch in place with Scotch Brand #33 plastic tape and some shoring. This type of patch must be inspected frequently, because it tends to slip or shift with the movement of the boat.

Holes above the waterline may be more dangerous than they appear. When the boat rolls, these holes may admit water into space above the center of gravity and reduce the stability of the boat. You can use either inside or outside patches on them. Inside patches may be made with pillows, seat cushions, or blankets, backed up with boards and shoring. On the outside of the hull, a good patch can be made with a board and a pillow or cushion that has a hole punched in the center. Pass line or marline through the padding and board and tie it securely behind the board. Then place the entire patch on the outside of the hull. Pass the line through the hole and secure it to a firm structure inside the boat.

A Homebuilt Collision Mat

The best preparation for hull damage is a collision mat, which is a canvas device secured over a damaged area of the hull so that water pressure helps keep it in place. Experience has shown that the best mat shape is triangular, so that it can be adapted to most of the irregular shapes of a yacht hull, including the bow. A single belaying line slung underwater, with two other lines secured on deck, usually will hold the mat in place. It may be possible to position the mat, without sending a person into the water, by maneuvering one holding line under the bottom from the deck. The mat should be about 4 feet on each side of the triangle. Heavy canvas of two thicknesses should be double-stitched together, reinforced at the corners, and have sheet-sized grommets in the corners. The collision mat is secured by lines (⅜ inch diameter) permanently attached to the mat corners. Each line should be long enough to be run under the keel of the boat, if necessary, and secured on deck.

Because of its shape and ready lines, the collision mat can be of great assistance in helping to protect a hull during a grounding, even when the watertight integrity of the hull is still intact. It can hold cushions, lumber, or other materials in place underwater when a grounded boat's hull is in danger of damage from rocks and other potentially damaging ground material, or hull abrasion from surf or current movements. Of course, buoyant material used to protect the hull must be lashed or held in place to prevent it from floating off.

Keeping the Bilge Dry

During a grounding all seacocks should be closed, with the possible exception of a raw-water engine intake valve (if the engine is to be used) and the seacock used for the bilge-pump through-hull opening. This is to prevent sand and dirt from clogging the openings and to help find the sources of any water coming aboard. Many automatic bilge-pump floats often will lock in the open position when the boat is heeled sharply. In that case, the boat should be pumped dry and the pump turned off "automatic," so it does not burn out. Watch for floating debris that can clog the bilge pump. If the bilge pump becomes inadequate or inoperable, then the engine intake hose can be disconnected from its through-hull fitting and placed in the bilge so it will suck up the bilge water and remove it through the exhaust. Again, watch for floating debris that could clog the engine water pump. These procedures should continue as needed throughout a grounding incident. Again, if aground on soft bottom, make sure bottom material is not being sucked into the engine cooling system. Keep an eye on the engine temperature gauge at all times.

Coast Guard Assistance

The Coast Guard can often assist in pumping your boat. They first will attempt to locate the source of flooding and reduce the flow of water into the boat. Their 41-foot Utility Boats (UTB) are equipped with an eductor, which can be used if weather and sufficient depth allow them to come alongside your grounded boat. Connected to a 2½-inch fire-hose, the eductor is placed either vertically or horizontally in the flooded area. Water from the Coast Guard boat's fire pump is forced through the firemain and out through the discharge hose. As this rapidly moving water passes over the suction opening, it creates a vacuum. The vacuum creates suction and pulls water up through the hose and over the side of the boat.

Both the 41-footers and the 44-foot Motor Life Boats (MLB) carry portable drop pumps. The P-140 pump can pump 140 gallons of water per minute, and it can be passed quite easily from one boat to another. If the Coast Guard vessel cannot safely approach a grounded boat, then the pump can be floated down to the disabled boat on a line strung between the two boats, with the pump sitting in its own water-tight container. The rigging for this may require that a messenger line be sent first to the grounded boat so that drawlines can be attached to the pump container for transferring the pump. If the current is favorable, it may be possible to float the pump down to the grounded boat via a mooring line rigged between the vessels. To operate the pump: (1) pull the handle to release the tension ring on the storage container; (2) lift the lid and open the plastic bag, then lift out the pump; (3) connect the hard green suction hose to the inlet on the pump (or eductor) and submerge it in the flooded area; (4) fill the gas tank (if not already filled; gas is supplied); (5) fill the pump housing with water; (6) pull out the green choke handle; (7) wrap the pull cord around the starter reel and pull, repeating as necessary until the pump starts; (8) as the engine warms up, push in the choke; (9) when pumping is complete or it is necessary to stop the engine, push the stop switch on top of the spark plug. Multilingual instructions are packed with the pump.

As mentioned in Chapter 1, Coast Guard rescue boats also carry emergency flotation bags, which provide approximately 500 pounds of buoyancy. As a general rule, one bag is needed for each 1,000 pounds of the disabled boat's gross weight to keep her afloat. The bags are used essentially to keep small craft from sinking, and no single small Coast Guard boat would carry enough of the bags to keep afloat a fully flooded heavy cruising boat. Nevertheless, this may be another available aid to resolving a bad situation.

CHAPTER 10

Towing

The decision to attempt to tow a grounded boat free should be made by the operator or owner of the grounded boat after considering all factors. It may be a more prudent decision, for example, to tow a grounded boat off a surf-swept rocky shore, with the distinct danger that the boat may sink near the shoreline once refloated, than to allow the boat to become flotsam from pounding on the bottom. The stage of the tide is important in this decision, as well as the extent to which the boat is being pounded or in danger of broaching. Where there is a great tidal range, it may be best to allow a holed vessel to continue pounding until it is either refloated on the flood (after temporary patching) or allowed to dry out on the ebb. Naturally, attempts should be made to keep the boat from ranging and from being driven farther ashore.

Once a boat has started to move, a dynamic coefficient is applicable—i.e., friction experienced in motion is far less than that found in static conditions—so keep a boat moving once she has started to move along the bottom.

Considerations Before Towing

As in any refloating technique, you need to determine the extent of hull damage before towing is attempted. If the grounded boat is holed, or seams have worked open on a wooden or metal boat, temporary repairs should be made to reduce leaking to a minimum. Besides the danger that the boat might sink just offshore, the weight of the water-filled hull may render the grounded boat immovable to the towing boat. The Coast Guard will not attempt to refloat a grounded boat if there is any doubt as to the vessel's ability to remain afloat (see Appendix B for Coast Guard policy).

If it is likely that the boat will remain afloat, then further action must be planned carefully to avoid unnecessary and excessive stress on the grounded boat's hull or towing rig. The following factors should be considered: Does the towing boat have enough power to do the job? Is the towing rig strong enough to take the static load? Are the fittings and hull structure of both boats adequate (using the strongest fittings)? What are the sea conditions? What are the tidal conditions? What is the existing weather? What is forecast?

Current

Regardless of the procedure used, the boat will be carried in the direction of the current. To counter this, the towing boat should secure the

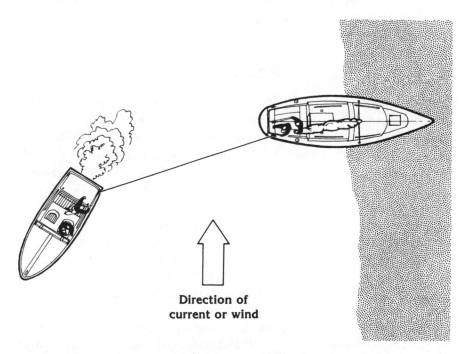

**Direction of
current or wind**

Figure 9. A towboat should steer to offset strong winds or currents in order to keep the grounded boat under control once she floats free.

towline forward of the stern or abaft its bow to increase maneuverability. Determine the set of the current and prepare for towing to counteract that force. (See Figure 9.) The grounded boat should usually have one or more anchors deployed to seaward to help prevent the boat from being driven farther aground.

Water Depth

Unless weight is removed from the grounded vessel, refloating should not be attempted at any lower tidal stage than that in which she went aground. Determine the water depth at the time of grounding (approximately the same as the boat's draft) as well as the time the depth will again be at least equal to that. Any premature effort will result in excessive strain on towing hardware and possible damage to the stranded boat. Obviously there have been many cases of boats being towed from a soft bottom soon after a grounding, but once the boat has settled firmly from an ebbing tide, it is risky to attempt to drag the keel over the bottom. Freeing the keel by shifting weight or heeling may help, however, if the procedure is carried out quickly.

Scouring

One of the greatest aids in refloating a stranded boat is the use of the scouring current from a powerboat that is available to assist in towing. This technique, which involves creation of a channel for the distressed boat, can be employed only when the boat is grounded in sand, mud, or gravel bottom, when the water depth permits the powerboat to work alongside, and when the boats are in protected waters. The 41-foot and 44-foot Coast Guard boats are ideal for this purpose.

Scouring a channel requires that the powerboat moor alongside the stranded boat amidships so that the powerboat propellers are directed diagonally down and under the grounded boat. Four preventer lines, two crossed and two straight, are used to link the two boats. The assisting boat commences to scour amidships, and, as the operation progresses, the powerboat is shifted forward and aft as necessary. This scouring action, combined with the pull of the assisting boat, will often refloat a grounded boat and keep her under control once she has broken free.

Tattletale Cord

Since sturdy towing lines are crucial to the success of a tow, it is important to know the safe working loads of the lines you are using (see Appendix A). But even though you know the safe working loads of your lines, there are so many variables that it often is impossible to operate within that range. Fortunately, the percentage of elongation of synthetic line under tension can be measured closely enough to determine when its safe working load is reached. A strain gauge, or tattletale cord, can indicate if an elongated line is nearing its breaking point. The tattletale cord is a bight of heavy cord or light line that is cut to a specific length, depending upon the type of synthetic line it will measure. (See Figure 10.) The ends of the tattletale cord are secured at a specified distance apart on the synthetic line, again depending on the type of line. As the synthetic line elongates under strain, the tattletale cord stretches with it. When the cord is drawn taut,

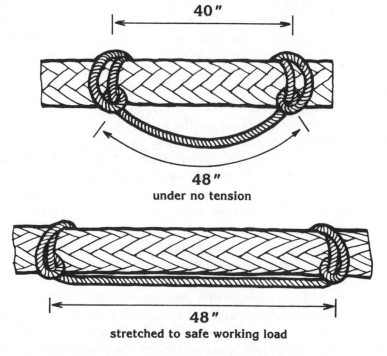

40"

48"
under no tension

48"
stretched to safe working load

Figure 10. A tattletale cord is an easy way to gauge strain on synthetic line. When the cord is drawn taut, the line has reached the percentage of critical strength roughly equal to its safe working load.

the line has reached the percentage of critical strength roughly equal to its safe working load. Use the table below to make a tattletale cord.

DIMENSIONS FOR TATTLETALE CORDS

Type of Synthetic Line	Length of Tattletale (Inches)	Length of Cord (Inches)	Critical Stretch (Percent)
Nylon (3 Strand)	40	30	40
Nylon (Double Braided)	48	40	20
Nylon (Plaited)	40	30	40
Polyester (3 Strand)	34	28	20
Polypropylene (3 Strand)	36	30	20

Transferring the Towline

In rough weather, it may be possible to pass a heavy towline only a few feet to a distressed boat. If the grounded boat is too far off, a messenger line must be used to pass the towline. The messenger is simply a length of light line that can be cast, propelled, or floated considerably farther than the towline alone. One end of the messenger line, of course, is attached to the towline. There are four types of messenger lines.

1. The heaving line is the preferred type of messenger. It is a light, flexible line with a monkey fist at the throwing end. (See Figure 11.) The line should be 15 to 20 fathoms (90 to 120 feet) in length. The other end of the line is secured to a towline with a clove hitch, a bowline, or two half hitches. If conditions permit, the best method of casting the heaving line is a leeward overhand heave (downwind). The range of the line increases if the wind is working with the line and the monkey fist.

2. The bolo is a heaving line made of shotline that has a toggle through the shotline about one fathom from the weighted end. The toggle extensions are grasped between the index and middle fingers of the throwing hand so that the line runs between the two fingers. With the toggle as support, the weighted end is swung overhead to obtain as much momentum as possible before the line is cast. The length of the line should be 15 to 20 fathoms, and the towline is secured to the other end, as described above.

3. Polyethylene float line, used with a ring buoy or life jacket, may be floated from upstream so that the line is carried by the current to someone on the distressed boat.

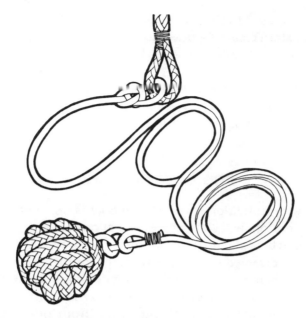

**Figure 11. A monkey fist is a time-honored, safe
weight for a heaving line. Here it is shown
attached to a heavy towline with a bowline knot.**

4. The 30-caliber Shoulder Line Throwing Gun (SLTG), used by
the Coast Guard, may be used successfully to pass a towline indirectly
when weather conditions are such that one of the other methods
cannot be used. It is often the only means of sending a messenger
during high winds and heavy seas. This SLTG should be used only by
trained personnel of the Coast Guard or commercial salvage units.

Deck Hardware and Other Gear for Towing

Adequate towing hardware should be available on both the towing
boat and the grounded boat. It is important to review your towing
equipment needs periodically, replacing or reinforcing fittings when
necessary. A fitting that breaks loose can become a dangerous missile.
A poor deck fitting can be the weakest point in the towing gear. Cleats,
bitts, and posts should be through-bolted with large backup plates to
take the strain of a tow. (Do not use deck cleats that are simply screwed
into place.) Towing lines may be rove through chocks to well-secured
sheet winches, or through positioned blocks (or strong tiedowns) to
the base of the mast. When the boat is being pulled off by the stern, a

bridle might be used to two stern cleats, thereby distributing the pulling load. But stern cleats are often used only for docking and are often too weak to handle heavy pulling, so be sure they are adequate before attaching a bridle to them.

Several fenders will be needed when towing alongside, as well as several docklines to hold the towing boat in place. These, of course, are normally carried aboard, but improvisation is possible.

The Straight Tow

A simple towing condition exists when a boat is only lightly aground, bow into the bottom and stern afloat, and allows for a straight pull off.

The towing boat should first determine the direction of the current, make sure the disabled boat is ready to secure the towline, consider anchoring in deep water at a safe distance, back down toward the stranded boat, then pass a messenger line to the boat.

When the towboat is positioned upcurrent from the grounded boat, the towboat might run past the stranded boat, paying out the messenger as it goes. The towline should be payed out sufficiently to ensure a good catenary (sag) in the line. Once the towing rig has been secured (see Rigging a Towing Bridle), the towing boat can start weighing anchor while moving ahead. This suggests that some form of winching or pulling gear is available on the towing boat, but if this is unavailable and extra hands are on the towing boat, then even they may supply the additional pulling power required. The stranded boat almost always can be pulled off best in the direction opposite to the course held when she first went aground.

Wrenching

When a towboat is assisting in a refloating operation, wrenching is another aid. It frequently happens that a grounded boat may be resting on a bottom type unfavorable for the scouring technique, or the water may be too shallow to permit another boat to work alongside the disabled boat. Wrenching involves pulling the grounded boat from side to side. Rotating the stranded boat breaks the grip of the bottom on the hull. The procedures are the same as those described above for the straight tow, with the exception that the pull is in a different direction; that is, the towboat alternately positions itself so as to move the grounded boat in one off-center direction, then repositions itself to move the disabled boat in the extreme opposite direction. This wig-gling effect, while pulling, is an effort to break her free of the bottom.

A Bow Pull from the Towing Boat

A bow pull is used when the wind and the current are offshore and there is no heavy surf. The towboat approaches the disabled craft bow-on, passes the messenger and towline from the bow, and then backs down to apply the tow. The towline is secured abaft the stem on the towboat for maximum maneuverability. One possible advantage of this method is that the screws of the towboat could be in deeper water. Another advantage may be that a stronger towing attachment (moor-ing bitt or cleat) may be located on the bow of the towing boat. The grounded boat may break free as it pivots.

Towing in Heavy Surf

Towing operations in heavy surf are, of course, very dangerous. As a general rule, only a towboat specifically designed for such conditions (such as Coast Guard vessels) should be used. And the Coast Guard will only attempt such operations where there is a risk to human life. Surf, breaking inlets, and bars all require extreme caution. Pleasure boats are not designed for most heavy surf conditions, so there is the ever-present risk of losing the towboat as well as the grounded boat.

The towboat attempting such a rescue normally looks for the lowest part of the surf line. Waves are timed until the series of breakers are determined. This indicates where the maximum and minimum waves can be expected, so the towboat can enter the breakers during a lull. As the waves pick up, the boat must be maneuvered to meet them head-on to avoid broaching. Surfing down the slope of a wave could cause the boat to pitchpole. The towboat skipper must make an on-the-spot decision as to how he can help the grounded boat. If the boat is towable, the approach should be made from upwind, maneuvering to the inshore side for passing the towline. If the disabled boat's prox-imity to the beach prevents approaching from the inshore side, it may be possible for the towboat to back toward the grounded boat, stand-ing ready to throttle ahead into incoming breakers. The crew aboard the stranded boat should be positioned as far aft and as low as possible; the helmsman should continue to steer, if he is capable. If the grounded boat is damaged (i.e., holed) or otherwise unsalvageable, then the tow should be aborted immediately and procedures should be begun for removing the crew.

Depending on conditions at the time, it may be possible for a towing boat to lower down a messenger line or a towline on a float through the surf. During such maneuvers, the towboat skipper should never allow his vessel to get broadside to the surf or directly beneath a plunging breaker (in the curl). Often a crabbing motion will work well, the result of taking breakers at slight angles off the bow. The towline should be kept short to help shelter the disabled boat from wave action. Towing in a surf is always risky business, and it cannot be recommended. It is a job for the Coast Guard or commercial salvors.

Rigging a Towing Bridle

The single-leg bridle is normally used to tow sailboats. The bridle is secured to the base of the sailboat mast (provided that the mast is designed to withstand the stresses of towing) by taking one round turn with the bridle leg around the base of the mast and securing the bridle to the towline with a shackle.

When the double-leg bridle (Y bridle) is used, it is rigged so that the legs distribute the pull on the deck hardware and the hull. Although no specific length is required, the legs must be long enough to prevent yawing. The breaking strength of the bridle legs must be equal to or greater than the strength of the towline. The Y bridle is secured to both bows or to the stern cleats of the towed boat or to both quarters of the towing boat. In all instances, bridles must be protected with appropriate chafing gear.

There are two other bridles that should not be used routinely. The cabin bridle runs around the superstructure of the distressed boat and the hull bridle runs around the hull. These two arrangements, considered to be extremely dangerous, are used only if a grounded boat has no adequate deck fittings (fittings not secured to the deck with through-bolts and backing plates). Both of these bridles require considerable line, which often is not readily available aboard small boats. Halyards and sheets usually are of too small a diameter to be used (see Appendix A, Minimum Rope-Breaking Strength). More important, control is difficult because of the amount of line required and the way it is placed around a boat for towing. Breaking strengths of the waist and tag lines (used to secure hull or cabin bridles) should be enough to endure static towing forces. There are many different ways to construct these two bridles, depending on the design of the sailboat to be towed, so it is difficult to recommend a safe method of constructing them. If one of these types of bridles is necessary to free a grounded sailboat, it is wise to use the rig only to free the keel, and not to tow the boat any appreciable distance. Once the grounded boat has broken free, a regular towline should be rigged for towing to safety.

CHAPTER 11

Salvage Rights

Every small-boat operator/owner should be aware of salvage rights—that is, rights of a salvor who rescues and saves a boat from wreckage, destruction, or loss. By law, as well as custom, sailors are obligated to do everything reasonable to help save lives at sea, but they are not obligated to try to save property. (There is no legal equivalent on land.)

Some sailors do have misconceptions concerning salvage rights. For example, if you accept a towline or assistance from a crew of another boat, that does not automatically entitle them to a salvage claim. The salvor must testify to the degree of the boat's danger, his risk, his time and effort, the degree of his success, and the value of the property. A court then will weigh these factors to determine the amount of any salvage award. An agreement may be made between a boat's captain and a salvor so that the salvor will have no salvage rights. A witnessed agreement to take a tow takes precedence over a salvage claim. Such a document may be in the form of a Lloyd's Standard Form of Salvage Agreement, long used in shipping circles, which is based on the longstanding "no cure—no pay" arrangement. This leaves the amount of the award to be settled later by arbitration. (Appendix C contains the wording of the standard contract.) This agreement, incidentally, need not be signed. It can be hailed between two boats (or ships) in front of witnesses and become binding.

In contrast to the principles of law applied ashore, admiralty law recognizes voluntary services to preserve the property of another. The purpose of a salvage award is to encourage the prevention of the destruction of property by appealing to the personal interests of the individual, as a motive for action, with the assurance that he will not depend on the owner of the property he saves for the measure of his compensation. Rather, he may appeal to a court of admiralty. This normally applies to ships in distress because of their value, but the law of marine salvage also can be applied to yachts. A marine lien is recognized where: (1) there is a marine peril to the property rescued; (2) the service is voluntarily rendered; and (3) there is success in whole or in part, or a contribution thereto. A grounding or stranding is considered a marine peril. Any salvage suit is subject to a two-year statute of limitations. It is heard in Federal district courts as admiralty action.

On the other hand, the rights of the owner of property lost are protected by criminal statute. According to 18 USC 1658: "Whoever plunders, steals or destroys any money, goods, merchandise, or other effects from or belonging to any vessel in distress, or wrecked, lost, stranded, or cast away, upon the sea, or upon any reef, shoal, bank, or rocks of the sea, or in any other place within the admiralty and maritime jurisdiction of the United States, shall be fined not more than $5,000 or imprisoned not more than ten years, or both."

Just the existence of a peril does not render the boat subject to salvage. When a boat's owner or operator rejects the services of another, there is no salvage situation. Salvors cannot force themselves upon a grounded boat against the will of the owner/operator. If he refuses them, compensation cannot be recovered by a salvor for assistance rendered against his will. This is true even if the boat sinks and the owner marks the location and commences recovery operations.

When a boat is abandoned by the owner, however, and is then salvaged by someone else, the boat becomes subject to a lien for salvage. The maximum liability of the owner to qualified salvors is the value of the boat after salvage, unless there is a special contract between the owner and the salvor. The term *abandoned* in salvage is the condition that exists when the owner/operator and crew have left a boat without hope of recovery and without intent to return. The boat becomes a derelict. Even then, the owner's property interest and title are not divested. In effect, the owner has lost the power to prevent salvage, and any salvage award will likely be increased due to the increased risk of total loss. A salvor has the right to take temporary possession of a derelict boat and can claim a salvage award for services rendered.

The Lloyd's salvage contract is considered universal in the marine world. Actually, such a contract is used infrequently in salvaging yachts, because the value gained by salvors usually does not justify the expense of large, professional, ocean-salvage efforts. Professionals usually reserve their resources for the potentially higher profits associated with salvaging cargo ships in trouble. The phrase, "insure it with

Lloyd's" has become known to almost everyone. The irony is that no one, ever, anywhere, has at any time insured anything with Lloyd's. It is not an insurance company at all, but rather an international market of insurance. It also is the world's foremost center of shipping intelligence. You insure *at* Lloyd's, not *with* Lloyd's, for its underwriting members are individuals who compete with one another and who carry their own profits and losses. The Lloyd's history goes back to 1689 in London. Their standard marine insurance form, provided to underwriters, was "revised and confirmed" in 1779 (having its roots in a 1523 Florentine policy) and has been substantially the same ever since.

The Lloyd's "no cure—no pay" salvage contract dates only from 1890, because the reigning monarch of England held all salvage rights before then. The agreement stipulates that the salvor would accept whatever remuneration a Lloyd's committee decided upon, with payment contingent upon the preservation of some part of the property in peril. This feature of the Lloyd's form is essential to any salvage agreement. To protect the salvor, the amount of payment was made subject to the decision of an arbitrator (if one was appointed). The arbitrator's decision can be appealed to an admiralty court, but few such appeals are made. As for the agreement itself, countless legal decisions have made its basic outline practically unassailable. Today a Lloyd's Standard Form is accepted as valid even if it is signed after the salvage service has been rendered. It can be written out in longhand on an ordinary sheet of paper, and some jurists hold that a radio message from an endangered vessel's owner, written out and recorded by the radio operator, would serve as a legal Lloyd's Standard Form. It is not by accident that Lloyd's coat of arms carries a single word as its motto. *Fidentia.* It means confidence or trust.

The Good Samaritan Rule

The wisdom of the U.S. Congress prevailed in the Federal Boating Act of 1971 when an unwritten agreement, often called the Good Samaritan Rule, was passed into law. The law freed people assisting a boat or boaters from any civil litigation. The section, similar to state laws that protect physicians and other trained individuals who aid victims at an accident scene, clearly states that aiding distressed boats or people on America's waterways is, in the first instance, a responsibility for those who are in a position to help, and, second, that they cannot be held liable for any civil damages as a result of rendering such assistance. The desired effect, of course, is to encourage people to go to the aid of distressed vessels and/or persons aboard them. Because of its obvious importance to would-be rescuers, the full citation is:

Section 16. RENDERING OF ASSISTANCE
IN CASUALTIES (46 U.S.C. § 1465)

(a) The operator of a vessel, including one otherwise exempted by subsection 4(c) of this Act, involved in a collision, accident, or other casualty, to the extent he can do so without serious danger to his own vessel, or persons aboard, shall render all practical and necessary assistance to persons affected by the collision, accident, or casualty to save them from danger caused by the collision, accident, or casualty. He shall also give his name, address, and the identification of his vessel to any person injured and to the owner of any property damaged. The duties imposed by this subsection are in addition to any duties otherwise imposed by law.

(b) Any person who complies with subsection (1) of this section or who gratuitously and in good faith renders assistance at the scene of a vessel collision, accident, or other casualty without objection of any person assisted, shall not be held liable for any civil damages as a result of the rendering of assistance or for any act of omission in providing or arranging salvage, towage, medical treatment, or other assistance where the assisting person acts as an ordinary, reasonably prudent man would have acted under the same or similar circumstances.

CHAPTER 12

Drying Out

Drying out a boat under controlled conditions is a common procedure in many parts of the world. Some British sailboats, equipped with twin keels, are moored in places where the boat grounds out on every low-water tide cycle. Many experienced boat skippers routinely dry out their boats to do bottom painting and repair work. It is also frequently suggested that drying out during an emergency grounding presents a good opportunity to scrub down the bottom and attend to certain underwater hull maintenance chores, such as checking through-hull fittings. Since weather and wave conditions frequently are not favorable, this may be an overemphasized favorable aspect of an unwanted grounding. Nevertheless, if it is realistic under the circumstances, it is a good technique for keeping the crew occupied while waiting for feasible tide conditions.

If you are aground on a falling tide and your initial refloating efforts have proved fruitless, you probably will *have* to dry out the boat. This presents few problems where there is a negligible tidal range, but it can have serious implications if the tidal range is, say, 13 feet.

Keeping the Boat from Ranging

Perhaps the most difficult aspect of a drying-out situation is control of the movement of the hull against the bottom. Abrasion can quickly hole a fiberglass hull. Wood seams can be wrenched open. Rocks or other obstacles can puncture or rip any hull. The contact with the bottom may be a pounding action, which, if severe enough, can destroy the boat as she goes over on her side.

Secure the boat with as many lines as possible so she will be neither driven farther ashore nor carried out to sea. This is to reduce ranging, or the movement of the boat against the bottom. If a boat is heeled shoreward, you may have to set two anchors toward deep water —one anchor from the bow and one from the stern. If this is not feasible, you might rig a midship-belayed anchor line. This will also help keep the boat from being driven farther ashore on the falling and the rising tides. Other lines should be directed from the disabled boat toward the shore, to hold the boat as still as possible and to keep her from floating free with the flood tide. Such lines may be secured to pilings, rocks, trees, anchors, docks, stakes, or whatever else is available.

Try to borrow additional anchors and lines if you run short. Use your sheets and halyards if necessary. This is the time to save the boat, not the rigging. Send someone ashore to purchase additional rope at a hardware store, farm store, or an auto parts store. Be innovative. Most yachts do not carry anywhere near enough ground tackle to handle complex drying-out situations.

Protecting the Hull as the Boat Settles

As soon as you decide that the boat is to be dried out, start preparations to protect the hull as it settles on its side. (See Figure 12.) Most of the material used to protect the hull will probably be buoyant, so it will have to be lashed in place to keep it from floating away. You can use floorboards, cushions, sails, fenders, tarps, and other suitable onboard material. Look along the shoreline for driftwood, planks, tree limbs (which you can cut), and other items that may be readily available. Ask local property owners for material you might use to protect the hull. For extra line, use halyards and sheets (if not already in use) and a collision mat, if you have one. Tarps may be rigged to hold protective material in place. Check the bottom for rocks and other hard objects that might puncture the hull, and move what you can out of the way. Make sure the rudder will settle clear. Dig out around it if necessary. All this may not appear orderly, but it should do the job.

One or more anchors may be set on the high side of the hull to help ease the boat down in a controlled fashion and reduce ranging. People in the water (wearing shoes) can push on the hull to help keep the boat from grinding or pounding excessively in the surf, depending on conditions.

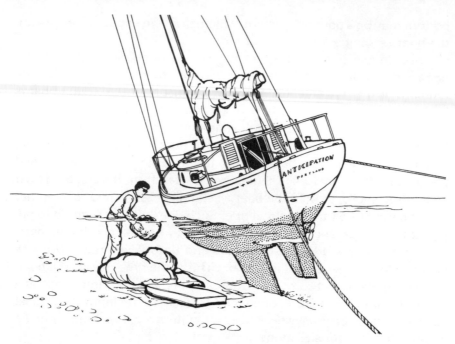

Figure 12. If a boat is aground on an ebbing tide, it is crucial to prepare to protect the hull as she dries out. Lines help to keep the boat from ranging.

Closing Down the Boat

Before the boat settles on her side, pump the bilge dry. Close all sea-cocks, not forgetting the engine intake valve. Shut down the master battery switch. Secure all loose gear by shifting it to the sole or the low side of the boat. Remove or seal batteries (tape tops, lash in place). Seal fuel and water deck pipes with waterproof tape.

Careening

The boat ordinarily should be careened, parallel to shore, to the high-ground side (usually the shore side) for drying out, so that the cockpit does not fill during the rising tide. If that is not possible, seal all cockpit openings (lazarette, lockers, companionway boards, etc.) with waterproof tape. A tarp may be lashed across the cockpit to prevent boarding waves from entering. Careening may be accomplished with a masthead line (see Chapter 8).

Holding the Boat Upright

It also is possible to make temporary legs to hold a boat vertical while drying out. (See Figure 13.) Some sailboats are known to flood with a rising tide after being dried out, making the use of temporary legs particularly appropriate. Production sailboats do not have this problem. One obvious hazard in rigging temporary legs is that a failure in the structure could topple the craft, possibly doing more damage than if you simply allowed the vessel to dry out. One leg is required for each side, plus a brace between them placed athwartships across the deck. Usually the legs are timbers, the main boom, or the jib-boom.

Lash the legs to the chainplates, turnbuckles, or deck stanchions; then lash the cross brace over the cabin (or deck) to the tops of the legs and to the mast. Secure guylines to the base of each leg, running the lines diagonally fore and aft from the base to cleats to hold the legs in place. If the bottom is soft, rig a base (floorboards, locker doors, planks) under the legs.

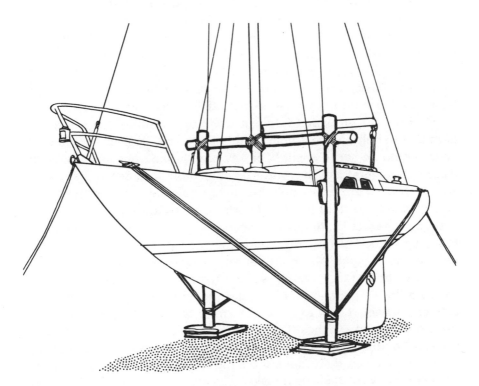

Figure 13. Experienced sailors sometimes fabricate makeshift legs to hold a boat upright as she dries out.

This technique can work quite well when the keel of an upright grounded sailboat sinks deep into a muddy bottom, so the keel takes the load and the legs simply keep the boat positioned. Legs can be difficult to place, however, and indeed may be hazardous if the sailboat has already taken on a list that cannot be corrected. It is possible to practice this technique when you are purposely drying out a boat for bottom maintenance. It is easiest to try it next to a pier or wharf.

Redistributing Weight

It becomes obvious that the centers of gravity shift as a grounded boat begins to heel. The center of gravity, that point at which all the downward forces of weight of the boat meet (or the center of mass of the boat), rises as volume is displaced. The center of buoyancy, that point at which the upward forces of support (buoyancy) meet (or the center of volume of the immersed portion of the boat), then will shift more and more to the heeled side. If the grounding occurred at high tide, the fall of the tide will result in a net loss of buoyancy and an increase in ground reaction (i.e., the bottom will seem to be lifting the boat out of the water). To assist a dried-out boat that is known to have difficulty in refloating itself without flooding through the cockpit (quite rare in modern sailboat design), or a boat that has settled in an unfavorable "downhill" position when dried out, try to remove or redistribute weight from the grounded side. Put strain on "righting" lines from the high side to help the boat float upright with a rising tide. The righting lines should be set to anchors or any handy fixed obstacles (such as trees or boulders), but they must be adjustable in order to maintain a strain. Often there exists only a delicate balance between the boat's natural ability to right itself or to take on the flood tide. Draining of fuel and water tanks, removal of gear, books, galley equipment, sails, tools, and much of the other items many boats carry will, of course, help remove weight. Also consider removing the boom and any furled sails, as these place weight in unfavorable locations. If needed, relocate the kedge and other ground tackle temporarily on the high side of the heeled boat to allow a strain to be placed on this side. Run lines to manned winches. Once the boat begins to lift with the tide without flooding, she can be expected to continue to lift to an upright position. You can then move the kedge and other ground tackle so they are ready for their next tasks.

Coping with Curious Crowds

Crowd control is an additional problem that a stranded sailor may have to contend with during a drying-out period. Unless you are on a deserted island, the spectacular sight of a boat over on its side, appearing to be wrecked, will draw observers from a wide area. In 1980 we went aground on a popular Maine beach in *Springtide,* our 33-footer, during a thick fog. Rapidly a crowd formed, perhaps 100 people, so we inquired as to how they all knew of the grounding. It seems that someone had called the local police to report the "wreck," and the call was intercepted by countless radio scanners and ham operators. The news was relayed instantly over a wide area, including the inference that wreck salvage was to be had for the taking.

Usually crowds do not just stand by passively and give gratis advice on how they would handle the grounding. Some may try to board or carry out their own ideas for aiding the boat, such as swinging on the halyards like Tarzan. It is common for people to board a stranded boat to look for items of salvage, in the honest belief that everything washed up on the shore is fair game. Teenagers will think the disabled boat a great place to have a party, often bringing their own beer to supplement whatever they might find on board. Men will shout orders to you, qualifying themselves by having had a hitch in some navy during the "big" war. Women will stand for hours in little groups to gawk and point at you, in between discussing the other news of the day. Parents will pose their children in front of your "shipwrecked" boat for photographs. The whole scene can be analogous to a circus, with you in the center cage.

For all practical purposes you can ignore all the amateur ungrounding advice heaped on you by bystanders. It may take precious time when you need it most, the source is questionable, and it can distract you from other activities you should be controlling, such as people trying to board your boat. If you have a hailer, use it to ask people to stay clear of the boat. Do not allow people to board the boat or even touch it. Be firm, be in control. If things get too uncomfortable, call the local police by VHF radio via the Coast Guard, who will relay the call. A crewmember might be able to go ashore and use a telephone to call the local police. Be sure the boat is attended at all times —through the entire 12-hour tide cycle if necessary. It is especially important to have a crewmember guard any equipment removed from the boat to lighten her. (Crewmembers should also tell the skipper what gear has been removed and where it is temporarily stored.) Check and recheck your holding lines to make sure no one has untied them, or worse.

Seeing your boat lying forlornly over on her side can be disheartening, but after you have recovered from the experience, you will probably wonder why you were filled with so much anxiety. In most cases, you will only have been inconvenienced, and because of it, you are likely to be a better pilot in the future.

PART THREE

PRECARIOUS GROUNDINGS

CHAPTER 13

Anticipating Danger

A review of serious grounding cases reveals that in some instances boat crews have had reasonable early warning that they were going to go aground. Usually this was during unfavorable weather conditions, such as off a lee shore, or when there was equipment failure, such as the loss of steering control. Under these kinds of circumstances, it may be possible to take action that can mitigate the effects of the grounding and aid in crew safety.

Use of Anchors

The most common last-resort technique for averting a grounding is to drop the anchor in order to try to hold the boat away from the shore or at least to buy some time. It is surprising how many skippers did not do this before going hard aground during adverse conditions, even though they had the time to do so. Apparently there is a strong desire to keep the boat running until the moment before impact. However, many fine boats have been saved from what appeared to be certain destruction by dropping one or more anchors in a timely fashion.

One 38-foot sloop, for example, that was driven close to a rocky lee shore during a gale, dropped her 35-pound CQR anchor in time to leave the yacht bouncing just 200 feet off a fierce beach surf. The keel whacked the bottom from time to time in the deep wave troughs, and life aboard was miserable, but the crew had time to deploy the liferaft and prepare to abandon the boat before the strain could part the ground tackle. Disaster was not meant to happen that windswept night, as a commercial salvage tug was able to lower a cable and pull them off. The anchor rode was ¾-inch nylon and there was 30 feet of anchor lead chain, 10 feet of which was ½-inch chain. The 2½-hour ordeal had distorted some of the links on the chain and had twisted the anchor flukes beyond repair, but it had held. The yacht owner believes that the anchor probably jammed into a crevice in bottom rocks.

It also may be possible to deploy one or more sea anchors to slow a boat in jeopardy of going aground. Sea anchors are canvas cones with the point open to allow for a controlled flow of water to pass through as they are dragged through the water to slow a boat's progress. If a cone-shaped canvas sea anchor is not available, then pails, anchors, or almost anything else that is handy may be dragged behind the boat to act as a sea anchor. Of course this would be an unusual circumstance, but most offshore sailors feel that it is hazardous closing on a lee shore during a gale while still a mile off. There may be time to mitigate the effects of the grounding. Furl sails, close seacocks, prepare survival equipment, prepare bow and stern anchors for release, radio your situation to the Coast Guard (they may arrange a land rescue effort), brief the crew on abandonment procedures, and so forth. It is also a good idea to collect supplies you may need once on land, since in remote places you may have to survive for some time before help is available.

CHAPTER 14

Deliberate Beaching

Many ships have been beached deliberately, and captains are still doing it today. In the sailing-ship era, vessels frequently were deliberately run aground when weather conditions were such that they might be forced aground anyway. In this way, the captains were able to select their landing places. Hundreds of such incidents have been recorded. Ferries on fire have been driven onto beaches to save passengers and crew. All kinds of commercial ships have been beached when faced with mechanical problems or serious leaking. During World War II, it was fairly common procedure to beach, bomb, or shell damaged ships, to be salvaged later. Monthly Coast Guard search-and-rescue reports include cases of damaged or malfunctioning commercial fishing boats being driven aground purposely to save the crew and boat. Yet many skippers do not even think of beaching their boats as a way to protect the crew or mitigate a bad situation.

Selecting a Beaching Location

If it appears that you are going to go aground anyway, you ought to try to pick the spot. In particularly nasty conditions, such a decision may make a big difference in saving the crew and/or saving the boat. Centerboard sailboats stand a better chance of surviving being driven up on a shore, of course, than do deep-keeled sailboats. Powerboat skippers need to consider their propellers. Nevertheless, the choices between, say, a sandy beach and a rocky shore might be available if the alternatives are investigated early enough. Obviously, beaching the boat will be a desperate decision, but oftentimes it is an intelligent one. If the boat survives, you will then need to follow basic ungrounding techniques.

A major problem with going hard aground at fast speed is that the keel, especially a fin keel, is subject to extraordinary torque, the impact of which can shear keelbolts and drive the keel back and up, thus fracturing the hull. The keel may become disengaged altogether from the hull. In a high, powerful surf, the boat may break up quickly and become flotsam. A full-keeled sailboat, with a long, sweeping keel line all the way aft, should handle a deliberate grounding more easily, being less susceptible to such keel dislocation. Keep the configuration of your keel in mind when selecting a beaching location. Unless there is some particular reason for wanting to drive the boat far up on the shore, given the circumstances at the time, slow the boat to a crawl before you strike bottom. Sea anchors, or something used as sea anchors, may be deployed to slow the boat.

Securing the Boat Once Aground

Once aground, the crew should act quickly to ensure crew safety and protect the boat, so have a plan in mind. Crew safety comes first, of course. Secure a bow line ashore with an anchor or tie it to a tree or other object (crewmembers can pull if no other solution is available) to keep the boat from floating off with a surging surf or rising tide. Other lines should be belayed to reduce ranging of the boat, which could grind or pound the boat open. Assuming the boat went aground bow first, consider setting a stern anchor to keep the boat from going farther ashore. Another possibility is to get a messenger line between the grounded boat and a boat standing off beyond the surf. An anchor line can then be attached to the messenger and an anchor may be taken out to be set. Or an anchor may be set off the shore and the bitter end of the anchor line can be floated down to the stranded craft. All other previously mentioned ungrounding principles apply to salvaging or mitigating damage to the stranded boat.

CHAPTER 15

Lifting Off and Digging Out

Many sailors neglect to consider digging and lifting as viable solutions for a grounded boat. These are everyday techniques for professional salvage men. Large stranded ships frequently have been refloated by having channels dug to and around them. Similarly, it may be possible to refloat a grounded yacht by dredging a channel to pull the boat into deeper water at high tide. Research reveals a surprising number of sailboats that have been abandoned permanently, never to sail again, because they were grounded (usually during particularly foul weather) too high to be refloated using normal techniques. If high and dry, a single small backhoe, a front-end loader, or a small bulldozer may do the trick. If such equipment is available, it may be possible to run a cable from the pulling machine on shore to an extra-large kedge (set in the water in the desired direction of pull) and back to the boat. A block will be necessary at the kedge. In effect, it is a two-part purchase that utilizes power from land machinery. U.S. Navy salvage teams successfully use such techniques to free their grounded vessels.

Some Professional Techniques

Following hurricanes or other severe weather, it is common practice to rig slings to a crane to lift grounded boats from where they were unwillingly deposited. They are then transported by land on flatbed trucks.

(Naturally this is a difficult, if not impossible, job if conditions are not tranquil.) There are cranes suitable for lifting virtually any boat, and they are land-based or sea-borne on barges. Their lifting capacities can be as high as 100 tons. Land-based cranes are quite readily available in most locations, but floating cranes often must travel from a distance, depending on where they are based or where they are currently in service. The Yellow Pages include listings for land-based cranes (look under Crane Service), and the district offices of the Coast Guard or the U.S. Army Corps of Engineers can supply information on floating cranes.

The processes of lifting off and digging out, of course, present problems of accessibility for the equipment. Unless you are familiar with the methods and technology involved, it is best to have the heavy-equipment operators address the problem. For example, they may be able to provide access from land more easily than you may think. Similarly, cranes on shallow-draft barges may be able to approach the stranded boat at high tide, extending the length of the crane to lift her off. Vacuum-type dredging barges can extend hoses considerable distances to dredge bottom material for a channel. A barge with high-pulling-power winches on its deck can set enormous anchors to hold the barge stable while its crew pulls a grounded vessel free from the bottom.

Helicopters

There is even the possibility of lifting a high-stranded boat, or parts of the boat (such as the mast), with a flying-crane helicopter. As bizarre as this sounds, it has distinct possibilities in unusual cases, provided the value of the boat warrants the effort and expense. In one case, a valuable 50-foot sailboat was forced high aground on an uninhabited New England island. The yacht, still in seaworthy condition, was declared a total loss by the insurance company, since salvage appeared impossible. She was sold for scrap to three sailboat owners, who hired a helicopter to fly out the mast and, later, the keel. With most of the weight removed from the vessel, it was possible to excavate a path to tow the hulk back into the water with a small tug. After a 25-mile tow to a boatyard, all the parts were reassembled and, in reasonably short order, she again became a much-admired yacht. The insured value was about $200,000.

The techniques mentioned here are not used as frequently as they should be by skippers of grounded boats. They just require some imagination. Be determined and innovative. Seek professional advice from those in the lifting and digging businesses, who may know little about sailing but may be able to make your day. Some examples of case-study applications of digging out and lifting off appear in Part Four of this book.

CHAPTER 16

Scuttling

To any sailor, deliberately sinking a perfectly good boat is unthinkable. But when the boat is aground, in imminent danger of being broken up by the surf, that may be one of your last remaining hopes of saving her to sail another day.

The purpose of scuttling, or sinking, a grounded boat is to keep it from sustaining damage from surf, current, and wave action. Settled hard on the bottom, the flooded boat will lose much of her buoyancy and the inside and outside water pressure will be equalized. The hull then will not move as freely as when fully buoyant, thus reducing damage to the hull.

Typically, boats are scuttled when they are pounding hard on the shore and in danger of being broken up. There are many variations on this theme, such as the huge sailboat that had drifted against a long cement dock during a full gale and was starting to break up from the pounding after all other efforts failed. (The boat was scuttled and later refloated and repaired.) There have been cases in which experienced skippers have scuttled their boats in deep water, just off the shoreline, to avoid almost certain destruction during particularly foul weather or loss of steering control on a lee shore. Often those yachts were raised from the bottom, repaired, and placed back in service.

While a serious step, scuttling does not have to be the frightful disaster that many envision. It is even possible for a scuttled boat to be refloated, cleaned up, and on her way with the next tide cycle.

Steps for Scuttling a Boat

Attach lines to the boat so that she will be held as firmly as possible (in all directions) against the bottom. The best way to do this usually is with anchors, but you can secure the lines to whatever is available, such as rocks, trees, pilings, or stakes driven into the ground. Sometimes you will have to use additional lines, such as halyards and sheets. You may need to borrow anchors and rodes from other boats, purchase rope at a hardware store, or use chain and steel cable from a farm or construction firm. If a Coast Guard boat is at the scene, it might have spare lines and anchors.

Set a kedge toward deep water to help pull the boat off when she is refloated and to keep her from being driven farther ashore. Bow, stern, and midship lines should be kept taut to keep the boat from moving with currents while full of water on the bottom. (See Figure 14.)

Remove what gear you can, but recognize that this is a real emergency and you probably will not be able to save everything you want to save. Do not bother with items that will not be damaged by water. Concentrate on electronic equipment. It is helpful to keep aboard a list of priority removable equipment. Open all hatches, portholes, vents, and anything else you can open so that the water can move freely

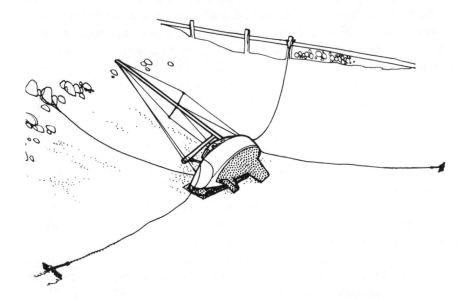

**Figure 14. A scuttled boat should be secured with lines
to reduce movement (and damage) as she rests on the bottom.**

through the boat, thus creating less movement when on the bottom. Close all seacocks to prevent clogging. Unclamp one or more hoses at seacocks and remove them from the fittings to allow the boat to flood. (These seacocks, obviously, would be left open.) Abandon the boat.

Refloating the Boat

As the tide recedes, the water will evacuate the boat through the open seacocks and you can board to prepare for refloating. You can also make emergency hull repairs at this time. If weather and/or wave conditions are still unfavorable, you may want to leave the boat flooded on the bottom for one or more additional tide cycles, until she can be refloated on a favorable tide and in calm weather.

The owner/operator of a scuttled boat can also hire professional salvage units to raise the boat. (Naturally, such arrangements should be made as quickly as possible following the scuttling to minimize further damage from amateur salvors or scuba divers seeking "treasure" or parts from the boat. It is usually impossible to keep such an event secret.) Usually the boat will be lifted off the bottom by a floating or land-based crane. Depending on water depth, divers may be used to secure lifting straps.

Scuttling may seem a strange way to save a boat, especially one you are very fond of, but the chances are that she will sail again another day. Scuttling allows you some choice in a bad situation, and in this case, stealing the boat's buoyancy works to your advantage.

CHAPTER 17

Basic Grounding Checklists

Since every grounding is unique (that is, no two situations are exactly the same), a number of options have been described in the last 16 chapters. At this point, a summary is in order, so the checklists below will serve as an easy reference tool in helping you determine what to do, how to do it, and when to do it.

For All Groundings

1. Issue PFDs to the crew; determine whether crew should go ashore (or be placed on another vessel).
2. Check for damage; administer damage-control measures.
3. Write down time of grounding (for computing tide levels).
4. Furl sails.
5. Be sure engine is idled or shut down.
6. Crew prepares kedge (largest anchor).
7. Crew prepares all other anchors and ground tackle for deployment.
8. Make soundings around boat from dinghy (or over the side if no dinghy is available) and mark them on a location sketch.
9. Make observations of current and wind.
10. Pump bilge dry.
11. Close nonessential seacocks.

12. Inform local Coast Guard station of the situation by VHF radio, if deemed necessary.

Basic Ungrounding Efforts

1. Deploy kedge(s) in the direction of deepest water and in direction of current and wind (if possible).
   a. Use heaviest anchor. More than one kedge may be set.
   b. Take kedge out as far as possible, using dinghy or floating kedge on life preservers, or other buoyant material, while swimming.
   c. Run kedge line to most powerful winch and put on a strain.
2. If boat is ranging badly in the surf, set port and starboard midship anchors.
3. Try short burst of the engine in reverse with full strain on kedge. Do not continue if boat is not refloated immediately (hard reverse engine can push bottom material around keel).
4. Set engine throttle at full ahead, with kedge holding boat in place, to try to scour bottom material from keel.
5. Determine if possible where the boat is in contact with the bottom, then shift weight (moving people and gear to one side) to try to break free.
6. Try heeling by placing people or heavy weights on a swung-out boom. Use a line from the masthead (i.e., halyard), if possible, to heel the boat.
7. Lighten the boat by moving people and gear to a dinghy or ashore. Pump the freshwater tanks dry (open lines and pump overboard with the bilge pump). Consider hand-pumping gas or diesel fuel from tanks. The fuel can be disposed of ashore or transferred to another boat. (Fuel oil pumped overboard would be a pollutant and would have little calming effect on surf.)
8. If boat is not moving dangerously with the surf, consider stationing dressed crewmembers in the water to push. All people in the water should be wearing shoes (cut feet would further complicate the situation) and PFDs.
9. If a powerboat is available (the bigger the better), it can be run back and forth to create waves, which will assist in dislodging the disabled boat. Make sure there is ample water to prevent the powerboat from grounding out.

Towing Checklist

1. Use the heaviest towline available (usually an anchor rode); transfer with a messenger line if necessary.
2. Make a Y bridle for the towed boat (two lines held together with a shackle or bowlines) to attach to stern cleats or stern winches. On a forward pull, make one turn around the mast, provided the mast can take such a strain.
3. Use a bridle if desired on the towboat to distribute the pulling load.
4. See that both crews are sheltered if nylon line is used (a rubberband effect results if something breaks loose).
5. Pull into the current and/or wind.
6. The towboat can deploy its own anchor forward, winched in hard, for additional pulling power.
7. Make sure that the pull is steady, not in running bursts, to avoid getting close to breaking strains on towing system. The grounded boat may help with bursts of the engine in reverse.
8. Try shifting weight (crew moving rapidly from side to side) during tow to break keel free.
9. The towboat can try pulling from different directions, i.e., wiggling the stranded boat.
10. Try a side pull if there is ample water depth. The towboat's propeller thrust will also have the beneficial effect of scouring sand and mud away from the grounded keel. The towboat can shift its position forward and aft on both sides of the grounded boat for maximum scouring effect.
11. The maneuvering towboat must be aware constantly of the danger of going aground herself, especially when there are strong currents and/or winds.

Drying Out (Depending on Conditions)

1. When hard aground on a falling tide, it is best to make immediate preparations to dry out the boat, before she heels too far over.
2. If possible, pivot the boat so she will come to rest on the highest bottom elevation, usually shoreward.
3. Careen the boat, by shifting weight or putting strain on a swung-out halyard, to the most favorable side of the boat. Side anchors may be used. This must be done before the boat heels too far to the least favorable side.

4. Place anchors to keep the boat from ranging in the surf and/or current.

5. Use padding to protect the hull from the bottom or obstacles.

6. Close all seacocks and hull openings after securing movable objects in the cabin (RDF, books, etc.). Seal cockpit lockers with waterproof tape. Turn off electrical master switch. Remove batteries or seal tops to prevent acid spill. Seal all fuel tanks to prevent spillage. Secure drawers and cabinets with tape if they do not have positive clasps.

7. If going ashore, take ample clothing, blankets, etc., to make your watch more comfortable.

8. If weather situation is not perilous, someone should remain aboard to tighten kedge/anchor lines, to keep rigging and gear secured, and to keep unauthorized persons from boarding the boat.

9. As the boat goes over on her side, make required adjustments to hull padding, rock removal, and so forth.

10. When the boat is dried out, inspect the underwater part of the hull. The hull may be cleaned or repaired while the water is low.

11. Deep, narrow sailboats may need some assistance in refloating, especially if mired in a muddy bottom. Anchors may be deployed in the direction of the high side and winched in with the flood tide. Lumber bracing on the low side, with people in the water exerting upward pressure, can also help provide the buoyancy to refloat a sailboat. Bailing may be necessary if water flowed into the cockpit with the incoming tide.

12. Be prepared to kedge the boat off the bottom once the water is sufficiently high.

13. Inform the Coast Guard of your situation (they will be receiving calls regarding your plight).

Scuttling

1. Safety permitting, remove valuable electronic and other equipment that could be damaged by water.

2. Place kedge in deepest water and set other anchors and lines to keep boat from ranging in the surf, current, and wind. Lines may be secured ashore, to docks, boulders, etc. Halyards and sheets may be used for such purposes.

3. Seal fuel tanks. Remove or disconnect and seal engine batteries.

4. Open all portholes and hatches to allow the water to move through easily when the boat is submerged. Remove at least one through-

hull hose from a seacock to flood the boat; close all other sea-cocks to prevent them from being clogged.

5. Abandon boat. The boat may be refloated on the next favorable tide, weather conditions permitting.

Other Considerations

1. Do not attempt to free a grounded boat at a tidal level less than that in which she went aground. Greater damage may occur than if she simply dries out and is refloated with the next flood tide.

2. Safety first. In bad surf or weather conditions, for example, it is probably best to move the crew ashore. Make this decision early to avoid compounding an already unfavorable situation. Deploy PFDs, liferaft, and other safety gear immediately. People in the water should be wearing shoes as well as lifelines attached to the boat.

3. Know when to abandon the boat. When there is no reasonable hope of salvaging the boat (as on a rocky lee shore in hurricane-force winds), leave the boat while there is still a platform to work from.

4. Do not risk the safety of other people or boats in an attempt to refloat your boat.

5. With the possible exception of Coast Guard assistance, make all decisions yourself.

6. Try combinations of ungrounding techniques. Knowing the principles, you may want to try other approaches, depending on the circumstances. For example, lines may be run fairly long distances to land, where a vehicle may assist in a tow, or hull-buoyancy tanks may be readily available ashore. Don't forget commercial assistance; large construction cranes have picked up many stranded yachts and trucked them home. Be imaginative and persistent.

7. Remember that the primary mission of the Coast Guard is to protect people. They have no responsibility for keeping your boat afloat.

PART FOUR

GROUNDING CASES

CHAPTER 18

Forty-Two Case Histories

The most reliable source of boating information is the U.S. Coast Guard, which issues annual summaries in the publication entitled *Boating Statistics.* Groundings are one of the 13 major types of statistical accident data collected through Coast Guard *Boating Accident Reports,* and groundings number in the hundreds each year. A relatively small number of fatalities each year are attributed directly to grounding accidents, but this is misleading because of the way the data are collected. Each report is categorized either by the reason that Coast Guard Search and Rescue was notified or by the severity of the incident. Thus, a grounding incident that also had a fatality when a person fell overboard might well be categorized as an overboard incident. Obviously, there are far more reported incidents that include groundings but appear under other categories. California has by far the greatest number of reported groundings annually (about one-fourth of the total), followed by Florida, Hawaii, and Michigan.

Other sources of grounding case histories are insurance companies, reports in boating literature, and interviews with crewmembers of grounded boats. For this chapter, all of these sources have been used. I am particularly grateful for several computer searches by various Coast Guard District Search and Rescue offices and insurance companies. In all official records, insurance records, and most individual interviews there is a request, or a requirement, that the information obtained remain confidential insofar as the right to individual privacy is concerned. To protect this privacy, no names have been used in the cases presented here.

A review of several thousand grounding cases reveals that the greatest number of reported groundings can be considered rather routine, with the Coast Guard having been informed only as a safety matter or for routine assistance. In most of these cases, in tidal waters, the boat was refloated by its own crew with a flood tide. Insurance companies know of these groundings because of claims. But the case histories also revealed a relatively large number of yachts lost because of groundings. Some of these stories are almost unbelievable. Boats have been run aground and destroyed under every imaginable condition and situation, and some are almost beyond imagination. Boats have been lost when grounded on a partially sunken freighter in the Caribbean, while stranded on a coral reef during a spring high off Mexico, when forced off course and rammed high aground on an uninhabited island during a gale in Rhode Island Sound, when the keelbolts gave way following a hard grounding along the Washington coast, and so forth. Storms, of course, take a large toll when they force boats aground, sometimes breaking them free from their moorings and carrying them considerable distances. The research shows that once on a lee shore during a gale, or worse, many boats are totaled, at least for insurance purposes. Groundings apparently are not newsworthy, so it is rare to hear of the serious groundings that take place daily on the nation's waterways. Similarly, research indicates that few groundings are cited in articles in the boating magazines, which seem to prefer instead to dwell on the more positive aspects of sailing.

The 42 cases included here were selected because they illustrate a successful technique or because they reveal errors of omission or commission. They are presented here so that they may contribute to the knowledge of appropriate ways to deal with similar situations. Every one of the thousands of recorded grounding cases is unique, but the techniques that worked or did not work in each of these cases are worth consideration.

Going aground can be shocking and embarrassing, but it need not be any more than an inconvenience if every effort is made to refloat the boat according to techniques described in this book. Groundings can happen to anyone—from the most experienced blue-water yachtsman to a dinghy racer—so be prepared, be innovative, remain calm and in control. Follow what you have learned in this book so that any future grounding incident will indeed be *only* an incident.

1

Cheoy Lee Offshore ketch, 31 feet, 10,800 pounds displacement, 3 feet 9 inches draft, aground on Oregon shore.

It was the worst storm in a decade, and the experienced crew of three had been caught close off a lee shore. The only jib halyard had parted earlier, leaving the ketch running on only a reefed main and mizzen. They could no longer make headway off the white sandy lee shore in the 60-knot winds and 20-to-25-foot breaking seas. The boat was taking an awful pounding, with the bows either buried deep in the water or high in the air, always in imminent danger of broaching. Without the jib they had little chance of working their way offshore. Dropping the anchors would bury the bows deeply and rob the boat of its buoyancy, inundating the craft. Moreover, they could not imagine the ground tackle holding long in the continuous onslaught of huge waves. To abandon ship in the inflatable liferaft seemed to mean being tipped over by the waves, to face the prospect of drowning, or to be upset in the mountainous frothy surf. They also could deliberately beach the oceangoing sailboat. They had few options. They agreed to beach the ketch, to drive her through the surf if possible, and to ground the boat at a point they could select. The 3-foot-diameter sea anchor was readied, its line secured to the mizzenmast. At 150 yards from shore, they selected a large sand beach between rock ledges, and the wheel was put hard over to run her aground. The sea anchor was released to slow her, lest she ram the keel free, possibly fracturing the hull. It was one hour after high tide. The wheel was lashed just before they approached the roaring surf, there being so much flying water that they would be unable to steer accurately beyond that point. By good fortune, the last wave going into the surf lifted the boat and, amid steep, white roaring water, deposited the yacht with a bump on her side on the beach, topsides on the high shoreline. Two more waves slid her a few feet up the beach, and there she stayed, later to be salvaged by land. The crew, bounced around in their life harnesses, were all saved.

2

S2 7.0 m. sloop, 23 feet, 3,600 pounds displacement, 2 feet 2 inches draft (4 feet 8 inches, centerboard down), aground on Lake Michigan sand shore, with some large rocks and boulders scattered about.

Driven aground with all canvas flying, the boat went even farther aground when the four relatively inexperienced crewmembers jumped into the water to try to push her off. A 28-foot sportfishing powerboat came along and offered a tow, which was accepted gladly. Using the powerboat's 250-foot, ⅝-inch nylon anchor rode as a towline, they decided to attach it to the bow of the disabled craft, and then around the mast, thereby turning the sailboat around as it came off the bottom. With the towline hanging loose, the powerboat gave full power to her twin diesels. The towline snapped taut, the sailboat's bow cleats shot into the air as they broke free, and the grounded boat jerked about rapidly, being dragged along the bottom at a fast pace. The hull of the sailboat whacked into a submerged boulder, cutting a 3-foot gash below the waterline. The powerboat charged ahead, dragging the hapless sailboat while her crew jumped for safety. Finally, the sailboat was heeled at 40 degrees with her rail awash. She sank in 25 feet of water, her tilted masthead just breaking the surface.

3

O'Day sloop, 25 feet, 4,200 pounds displacement, centerboard model with 2 feet 3 inches draft up and 6 feet down, aground on mud bottom in southern Chesapeake Bay.

When the boat was driven hard aground under full sail with four young men aboard, the partially lowered centerboard was forced into the fully retracted position. With sails lowered, they tried heeling the boat (with two of the crew on the end of the extended boom while kedging) to no avail, because the round bilge simply sank into the mud when heeled. A small powerboat with a powerful outboard engine attempted first to create waves to break the sailboat free from the suction of the mud, and then, second, to tow the stranded boat into deeper water. Neither attempt proved successful. They could remove little weight from the boat except themselves. At high tide the entire crew of four went into the water, but they could not break the boat free. Finally they decided to try to turn the boat around, using a combination of techniques. The kedge line was belayed to the bow, as was a towline to the powerboat. One crewmember manned the kedge line aboard, which was directed to a sheet winch through a rigged bow block. One of the experienced sailors manned the sails. Two crewmembers, wearing shoes, went in the water to push at the bow. On command, all efforts were executed, and, ever so gradually, the boat came about. Once she had broken the suction of the mud bottom, they were able to slide the two tons of weight into deeper water and continue on their way. The combination of techniques had done the job.

4

Ericson sloop, 27 feet, 7,000 pounds displacement, 3 feet 11 inches draft, aground on central California sand and rock shore.

Anchored in a small cove, the cruising sailboat was caught unaware by a swiftly moving squall, followed by foul weather. The 45-knot gusts slammed the boat into the base of a high rock cliff, holing the hull. The boat sank in 5 feet of water, the masthead against the cliff. The crew of three had scrambled up on a ledge about 10 feet above the water, wet but safe. The waves were building, moving the boat a foot or two with each wave, but the tide was ebbing. The sandy bottom at the stern soon had only 4 feet of water, so the two men decided to set an anchor from the stern to reduce the movement of the hull against rocks at the base of the cliff. The effect of this was noticeable immediately. They boarded the vessel and took two settee cushions to wedge between rocks and the hull of the grounded boat. As the tide receded, to a low of about 18 inches, much of the water in the hull drained through two jagged 8-inch holes. The boat was moved off the ledge rocks by tying the jibsheet and the mainsheet to the spinnaker halyard. The bitter end was run through a block lashed to a rock abeam the high side of the hull (i.e., in the direction of the pull) and winched in with the main halyard winch. The crew had found pieces of lumber on the beach, so they cut them with a hacksaw and made jury hull repairs by placing pieces of the wood over the holes inside and out. A single bolt held the wood together and in place for each hole. Clothing was cut up for gaskets and the boat was pumped dry. Bow and stern kedges were set amidships, away from the cliff, and drawn taut. As the waves of the flood tide raised and lowered the boat, pounding the keel on the bottom, they winched in on the kedge lines, which had been led via blocks to the sheet winches. All halyards and sheets had been stripped to be used for belaying lines from the boat to shore. One man remained on board as the sailboat began to float, winching her into deeper water amid the building surf, and later beyond. Two crewmembers ashore held lines (made from halyards, sheets, docklines, and spare lines) that were attached amidships. Once the yacht was in the best location in the cove to ride out the storm, the shore lines were belayed to boulders. The crewmember aboard floated downwind on the inflatable dinghy, through the surf, to land. The sailboat rode out the storm and later was rerigged to sail into the nearest harbor for more permanent repairs.

5

Hinckley Pilot yawl, 35 feet, 13,700 pounds displacement, 5 feet draft, aground on rock bottom on the Canadian New Brunswick coast.

Two Baltimore couples, enroute to St. John Harbor, were forced close to a high-surfed rocky lee shore during a strong August gale. When 300 yards off, with mizzen, storm main, and roller-reefed jib set, the skipper ordered sails furled and the 35-pound plow bow anchor readied for lowering. He no longer could hold against the 52-knot winds and high breaking seas. The 4-foot-diameter sea anchor attached to 200 feet of ½-inch nylon line was also prepared, and, as he brought the bow into the wind, let go. The strain was tremendous, but the yacht continued to close on the lee shore. Next the bow anchor was dropped and 300 feet of ⅝-inch-nylon rode payed out. Seventy-five yards off the surf, it took hold, broke loose, then held again. The captain, in evaluating the situation, felt he had run out of options to save the boat and concentrated on crew safety. The boat was pitching so badly that the ground tackle could not be expected to last very long. The keel was pounding the rock bottom when in deep wave troughs. The skipper decided that they had to go through the surf in the liferaft. The inflated liferaft was belayed close to the stern. A 300-foot anchor rode was rove through a block lashed to a stern cleat and attached to the liferaft bow ring. The bitter end and the balance of the line were placed in the raft. Crewmembers boarded the raft and lowered themselves toward the huge surf under some control. As they entered the surf, they released the line and the raft went flying onto the shore in a topsy-turvy fashion. Three of the crew sustained minor injuries and cuts as they scrambled to safety, and local people arrived to assist. The boat soon broke its bonds and was destroyed. An inquiry by Canadian officials concluded that the disastrous grounding was virtually inevitable and that crew safety should have been, as it was, of paramount concern. The evacuation technique was unorthodox but effective.

6

Mariner sloop, 28 feet, 7,500 pounds displacement, 4 feet 5 inches draft, aground on New Hampshire rock ledge at high tide.

By the time the crew of three women had tried motoring off the rocky bottom, the 10-foot tide had started to ebb and had wedged the keel firmly aground, the light wave action pivoting the sailboat from side to side. The large 22-pound bow anchor was brought aft with its rode and lowered into the dinghy, which they had been towing. One of the women rowed out to deep water, as far as the kedge line would allow her to go, before cutting the light line that held the kedge in place at the transom of the dinghy. On the return trip, she took new soundings with a leadline, making depth notations on a paper pad. Selecting the starboard side as the least rocky for drying out the boat, the women hiked out on the starboard shrouds while the woman in the dinghy pulled on the bitter end of a halyard. As the boat began to settle on her starboard side, they ran out a second anchor forward and off the port bow (weather direction) to secure the boat further. Padding was prepared to protect the hull as she settled on the rocks. Two tarps, a floorboard, and a settee cushion were lashed in place with sheets and spare light lines. When the boat was heeling 40 degrees, two of the women waded in the cold water, fully clothed and wearing shoes, to make final adjustments to the gear used to protect the hull and add several drift-wood logs and timbers found on the shoreline. One woman stayed on the boat to take the first watch, while the other two rowed ashore to seek shelter, knowing the ordeal would last at least 12 hours before they might unground the boat. The crewmember aboard tended to other drying-out chores, securing gear, pumping the bilge, and so forth. As the tide flooded, however, the boat had somehow become wedged between boulders and rock outcroppings, and water started to flood the cockpit. With quick, efficient work, the three women reset the kedge and bow anchors as far off the high port beam as they could, reeving the lines through rail-lashed blocks to the sheet winches. Full strain was put on the anchor lines, but still the boat remained on her side, taking water over the lee coaming. In chest-high water, two of the experienced yachtswomen rigged a long timber lever, putting their full weight on the outboard end, with the third sailor tending the winches, and the combined efforts broke the heavy boat free. When listing at only 20 degrees, they again reset the anchors as kedges, but this time both were off the stern. Knowing the forward part of the keel was on a shelf, they moved all the weight they could, including themselves, to the stern. At dead high tide she was kedged off into deep water.

7

Bristol ketch, 32 feet, 11,300 pounds displacement, 4 feet 3 inches draft, aground on a sandy North Carolina barrier island.

The two couples and one child aboard initially considered this ground-ing more of an inconvenience than a serious emergency, because it was at half water on a flood tide. The keel was barely touching, so they waited for the tide to break them free, the sails luffing. Once free from the bottom, they set the sails in an attempt to run off the long sand island, several miles from the mainland, in a 20-knot wind. In doing so, somehow they were set farther aground near high tide. As the 4-foot tide dropped, so did the sturdy cruiser, on her starboard side with a foot or so of water still around the craft. The surf built up as an offshore gale moved toward the stranded boat. At high tide, in a heavy surf, they attempted to kedge the boat off, but the force of the pounding 4-foot waves and the 35-knot winds prevented them from moving the boat far, eventually even slamming the boat more firmly aground when the kedge broke out. They called the Coast Guard on the VHF radio to ask for assistance when it became evident that the yacht could not be moved. When the boat started to flood through the companionway from the constantly flooded cockpit, the crew was moved to higher ground by a Coast Guard helicopter, which momentarily landed near the boat just before the full force of the gale arrived. The abandoned sailboat was damaged beyond reasonable repair and was never fully salvaged.

8

Fisher motorsailer, 34 feet, 19,500 pounds displacement, 4 feet 9 inches draft, aground on mud bottom in San Francisco Bay.

Moving ahead rapidly under power in fog with a crew of two, the boat was put hard aground near high tide. She was not far off a buoyed channel. Kedging did not free the craft and, as the tide ebbed, she sank deep into the soft mud bottom. On the next high tide, the yacht seemed to be captured by the bottom even more firmly, leading the skipper to speculate that shifting bottom material carved by currents was entrenching the boat. While seeking commercial tug assistance, the skipper recalled that during his hitch in the Navy, some 25 years earlier, salvage crews often used inflatable buoyancy bags to raise small vessels. Moreover, Navy salvage crews in training were often searching for appropriate exercises. A taxi ride to the U.S. Navy installation confirmed that, indeed, there was a unit in the Bay Area trained in such marine salvage work. But, as much as the Navy team wanted to practice their salvage skills on the yacht, there had to be a reason to use government men and equipment for private salvage work. The convincing reason was that because the boat was stranded near a channel buoy, she was a hazard to navigation. Soon a team of enthusiastic Navy salvage men appeared in three small boats loaded with gear. As one team of divers took down a compressed-air hose to burrow a trench under the keel, another team prepared to inflate four huge rubber buoyancy bags. Two slings were worked under the keel, where holes had been blown with compressed air, to be belayed to two partially inflated buoyancy bags on each side of the vessel. The bags were then inflated by a compressor mounted on one of the Navy craft. The grounded boat was lifted clear of the bottom in a jiffy and taken to deeper water.

9

Cape Dory cutter, 30 feet, 10,000 pounds displacement, 4 feet 2 inches draft, aground at night on rocky bottom near the Connecticut coast.

The cruising couple, in taking soundings, was surprised to find that deeper water lay ahead of the yacht, and not in the direction from which she had come. This was attributed to the fact that the boat had been heeled about 20 degrees in a 15-knot wind when she went aground, thus giving her reduced draft. Kedging while careening the boat at high tide was ineffective. For some distance astern of the grounded boat, the water was fouled with outcrops of rock and boulders, making the approach from that direction hazardous for a towboat. Directly ahead, toward the shoreline 200 feet away, was a narrow channel where the boat could possibly be worked along, but rock obstacles so restricted maneuverability that it would be hazardous for a towboat to operate there too. The sturdy sailboat, it was discovered, was virtually surrounded by obstacles that would endanger salvage boats. A kedge set off the bow did not budge the boat, apparently because the angle of pull forced the boat farther into the bottom. They needed a horizontal pull to slide off the rocks. The skipper took the dinghy ashore and carefully examined the predicament from there. He decided to attempt a land tow. From a Coast Guard 41-footer on the scene he borrowed a 1-inch towline and a large snatchblock. The towline was secured to the mast base on the disabled pleasure boat and then taken ashore to be rove through a block that had been secured to a large tree directly in line with the desired towing route. The bitter end was then taken 35 feet and secured to the towing ball of a volunteered pickup truck. Ten teenagers from the gathering crowd volunteered to act as ballast in the truck bed. Crews in small boats were asked to line the channel to keep the yacht in place once she came off.

A helpful community spirit prevailed. Everyone genuinely wanted to contribute something to the ungrounding and the delicate task of wending the boat through rock hazards back to her proper element. The cooperative effort succeeded, and the cutter crew was soon happily on the way, wiser for the experience.

10

Albin Vega sloop, 27 feet, 5,100 pounds displacement, 3 feet 10 inches draft, aground on a sandy Pacific shore in Panama.

The sailboat had been shoved hard ashore on a high tide during foul weather while enroute to San Diego. For three days, the crew of two had been trying to extricate the boat without success, essentially because the boat had been transported about 300 feet across an almost flat bottom by the force of the storm waves. The boat was stranded high and dry at low tide, forcing the couple to set up camp on the jungle shoreline. Indeed, they suspected that their options to refloat the boat were nonexistent. A small native village was two miles away, but there were only a few small fishing boats and fewer motorized vehicles. Most of the heavy work was done with a couple of tractors and oxen teams. They decided to make a final attempt before they abandoned their floating home and made their way back to the United States. They would try to drag the small yacht back to deep water. They had little to lose at this point. They first had to strip the boat of all removable weight, a job much more difficult than first anticipated. They traveled the 200 feet across the sand to the jungle edge dozens of times, usually towing gear on branches lashed together, much as American Indians used to do. They lowered the mast with a block-and-tackle arrangement and dragged it to the shoreline, clear of high tide. They moved a ton of gear and equipment ashore. They drained fuel and water tanks and removed the rudder. Finally, after three days of labor, all that remained was the hulk of the hull and cabin, perhaps two tons of it. In the village they contracted with the owner of an oxen team for his services, bartering some goods for part of the payment. After long timbers were cut and lashed together to act as a skid, the tow began. Progress was dishearteningly slow at first, but after two days, they had moved the boat 150 feet across the sand. On the third day, they wallowed through a foot of water at low tide to a point where the boat would float with the rising tide. There she was anchored while they returned to the village to recruit the operator of a small fishing boat to transport their provisions and gear out to the boat at high tide. The final item was the mast, which two fishermen and the couple lifted aboard and stepped in the cabintop tabernacle. Two weeks after the stranding, the couple resumed the voyage.

11

Ericson sloop, 39 feet, 19,000 pounds displacement, 5 feet 11 inches draft, aground in August on a Gulf of Mexico Mexican lee shore as a result of Hurricane Allen.

Winds of up to 120 m.p.h. forced the yacht into the inundated forest floor adjacent to the beach—only possible because of a 15-foot surge. The site of the wreck was inaccessible by vehicle, and the boat lay holed on her port side 175 feet from the normal waterline. The uninsured yacht was declared unsalvageable and was abandoned by the owner. Months later, a San Francisco woman sailor heard of the situation and purchased the boat for 5 percent of its market value. After establishing a base of operations in an inexpensive hotel in the nearest village to the stranded boat, she hiked through the junglelike forest to the boat. Her initial sight of the wreck was discouraging. The two-year-old boat was partially full of mud and sand and had two 6-inch holes in the hull. The mast was unstepped and tangled in debris, the hull was battered and partially covered with logs and other material that had floated up with the storm. Soon, however, the woman had hired local workers, who were able to repair and clean the yacht in a few days. The boat was hauled into a vertical position and blocked with a powerful portable winch carried four miles overland from the nearest road.

But there remained the problem of moving the boat 50 feet out of the forest and across the wide beach to be launched. It occurred to her that a perfectly normal way to move the rig would be on a railroad similar to those used by many marinas. A clever bit of investigating and negotiating resulted in the loan of tracks and railway wheels from a local railroad terminal. For two Saturdays she was able to hire a work crew of 25 local men and women, at very reasonable wages. They prepared a sand ramp and then hauled in (from a rented truck) and set track on ties cut from forest trees. Next they used several small hydraulic car jacks to move the yacht up to a specially constructed log cradle on the railroad wheels. Several long lines were attached to the cradle, and the work crew pulled the boat down the temporary track and into the water at low tide. Later, the new owner sailed away with a boat that had cost her only $9,500.

12

Columbia sloop, 29 feet, 8,500 pounds displacement, 4 feet 8 inches draft, aground on a Long Island Sound sand beach.

The sturdy racing/cruising sailboat was caught in a September gale, the force of which had caused the port masthead shroud to part. Fearful of losing the spars, the crew of two women and one man remained on starboard tack, keeping tension on the starboard shrouds. As the 8-foot waves increased to 12 feet, it was clear that the boat could not indefinitely continue beating in its disabled condition. Only 100 yards from shore, the crew elected to beach the boat through the huge surf. Dragging a sea anchor to slow the boat, they entered the roaring surf perpendicular to the beach, but a following wave slammed the yacht broadside in a broaching, knocked-down position. Successive waves skidded the boat high onto the beach, the storm surge providing 4 feet of water above normal. The crew, aided by people on shore, was saved. The sailboat, lying on her port side, the mast pointing toward high land, was secured from further movement by two anchor lines and one shore line. Two days later, at low tide, the boat was 135 feet from the edge of the water, resting against a sand dune. The nearest road was three-quarters of a mile away across rough terrain. The boat was repaired and made seaworthy, but there was still the problem of refloating her. Crane equipment could not be brought in because of inaccessibility, but a small tractor was able to reach the site. Ten people assisted as the boat was raised on her keel, with the tractor pulling on towing cables, and blocked in place. One of the owners had at one time been in the U.S. Forest Service, and he suggested sledding the boat back into the water, much as logs were formerly sledded out of the forest. A sled was constructed from heavy timbers and the boat was jacked into a cradle bolted to the sled. To gain the tremendous pull needed from seaward, they hired a small tug with a powerful stern winch. The tug was anchored 200 feet off the shore with three huge chained anchors, and the winch cable was taken to the sled. Foot by foot, the winch pulled the heavy boat toward the water. Four hours later, she sat in 4 feet of water. At high tide, the crew sailed away happily.

13

Bristol sloop, 33 feet, 13,000 pounds displacement, 6 feet draft, aground on the mud bottom off a Rhode Island peninsula.

The sloop had been sailed hard aground one hour after high tide with four persons on board (two couples). A normal drying out was considered infeasible because of the craft's exposure to the surf. Gale warnings had been announced earlier and the seas were beginning to build. The quick-thinking skipper had the crew prepare the available two anchors to be taken aft in the dinghy for kedging. He then put out a call on the VHF radio for anyone in the immediate vicinity. Two boats responded, and he requested ground tackle. In addition, he was able to hail a large powerboat, which was standing off 200 yards. In short order, the bitter ends of three additional anchor lines were brought to the stern, their kedges already having been set in a fan pattern off the stern. The crewmembers took the five kedge lines to the anchor, sheet, and halyard winches and applied full strain. As the seas became higher, they lifted and dropped the boat, each wave allowing the crew to crank in more kedge line. She came off the grounding under control and all involved were quickly on their way, well before the storm had time to materialize appreciably.

14

Wooden schooner, 49 feet, approximately 47,000 pounds displacement, 8 foot 6 inches draft, aground in central California harbor.

The older sailboat was forced aground on mud bottom in the outer harbor when she lost steering control while under full sail. After three weeks of trying to extricate the boat himself (without commercial salvage help), the owner sold the boat at a modest price to a couple without sailing experience. The boat was not a hazard to navigation. At high tide, she was about 2 feet short of sufficient water depth to be refloated, and she was entrenched solidly in the mud. The young couple had little interest in sailing the boat, intending to move her and use her as a floating home, and they had little money. The boat leaked so badly that small bilge pumps could not keep up with the inflow, which soon filled her and forced her even more solidly into the soft mud. The couple sought and received all kinds of advice, professional and amateur. They liked the idea of flotation bags, but, after receiving estimates, found commercial assistance beyond their economic reach. Then the young wife suggested using plastic garbage bags to add buoyancy. She reasoned that lots of bags, all contributing their share, eventually might do the job. Her husband, the recent recipient of a master's degree in mathematics, calculated their requirements and they set to work. The greater number of garbage bags, inflated with a small gas-powered compressor, were positioned on the outside of the bow and the stern quarters, where rope slings (placed by a skindiver friend) held them in place. It took two weeks to secure almost 250 bags, presenting a weird and entertaining sight to local observers following the work. For a small fee, the couple rented two large gas-powered water pumps from a local construction company. Finally, they mustered six small-powerboat operators to tow, figuring that six small tows equal one big tow. As the last garbage bags were inflated, and the pumps squirted huge volumes of water over the side, and the six small powerboats attached to six long lines ran up their engines, the schooner began to move. The beer party aboard the schooner, later tied to a dock, was still going strong at midnight. And the couple figured they had a supply of garbage bags that would last them at least five years.

15

Finnsailer cutter, 35 feet, 20,000 pounds displacement, 5 feet 2 inches draft.

A woman charter/delivery captain was hired to deliver the yacht from St. Andrews, New Brunswick, Canada, to Annapolis, Maryland, in November. Enroute she encountered a fierce gale off the rocky eastern Maine coast. Being forced onto a lee shore by the 55-knot winds, she opted to enter a large cove on an island, hoping for some respite from the storm, but she found little protection. For three hours, she fought to keep the yacht off the solid-rock lee shore inside the cove, becoming exhausted in the process. It was clear that the storm could not be expected to abate soon, and she was slowly losing what little searoom she had. When about 100 yards off the shore, she decided to scuttle the cutter, hoping to keep the boat from becoming flotsam. In a display of outstanding seamanship, she set both roller-furled foresails, ran the engine full ahead, and took the boat into the weather and into the middle of the cove. With the wheel lashed, she deployed the liferaft off the stern, cut two through-hull hoses to flood the boat, opened all portholes and hatches, dropped the sails, boarded the liferaft, and abandoned the boat. Fortunately, she survived the high-breaking surf with only minor injuries and was located by the Coast Guard, several hours later, in a summer house on the island. The following spring, the yacht was salvaged commercially from 65 feet of water, was repaired locally, and was sailing again before the end of the season. The greatest amount of damage was in the interior—the hull and spars remained intact but required refinishing.

16

Flying Dutchman cutter, 35 feet, 19,000 pounds displacement, 5 feet 2 inches draft, aground on a half-tide sand/rock shoal off Vancouver Island, Canada, during foul weather.

The yacht had struck the submerged shoal while making 8 knots with only a storm trysail set in the strong gale. The boat was heeled to port, preventing the couple aboard from making emergency outside hull repairs to an underwater hole in the port bow. The damaged area was under the V-berth and inaccessible. Temporary inside patching would only stem part of the water inflow, and the water soon was a foot above the floorboards. It was two hours before high tide, at which time the boat would be covered by the 11-foot tidal range. The gale had taken them off course in the Juan de Fuca Strait near Vancouver Island, and they could not see land. The couple elected to abandon the grounded craft immediately, using the time available to make an orderly departure. They radioed a Mayday message to the Canadian Coast Guard, suggesting that the U.S. Coast Guard, on the other side of the wide strait, also be informed of their predicament. They provided their Loran coordinates and said they would be near the boat. As the boat filled, they gathered ample gear to survive the storm in their inflatable liferaft. After they detached the main rode from the anchor and secured it to the liferaft, they boarded the raft with their survival equipment and fed out 300 feet of rode (which had been coiled in the raft). The raft floated quite comfortably at the end of the line attached to the boat, which soon rolled over on her side and sank. The rescue boat knew just where to find them.

17

Wellcraft Nova powerboat, 26 feet, 5,200 pounds displacement, 2 feet draft, aground on a sand-and-rock Northern California beach.

The boat was beached at low tide while making substantial headway, striking a rock that punctured a 6-inch hole in the hull. The local police found that the two men and one woman aboard were under the influence of alcohol. In an effort to save the boat, the police secured the services of a large tow truck, running its towing cable 180 feet down the beach to the disabled boat. They used seat cushions, shored with driftwood and planks, to stem the flow of water from the hole in the bottom. But the 3-foot surf and the flooding tide continued to pound the boat. The police feared that dragging the boat over the rocky beach would hole her beyond repair, so they radioed their headquarters, which in turn contacted a local logging company. Soon a large, loaded logging truck rumbled across the beach to the site. One lumberjack operated the "cherrypicker" (the truck-mounted log crane), swinging long logs to a man on the ground, who promptly cut them in half with a chainsaw. The cherrypicker operator skillfully arranged the logs in front of the boat, leading up the beach. Then the tow-truck operator slowly pulled the valuable boat up the beach on the rolling logs, ahead of the rising water, and the lumberjacks recovered their logs as the pull proceeded. Soon the boat had been transported beyond tidal flood waters, later to be removed from the scene by a specially equipped tractor-trailer rig. The court assessed the boat owner/operator all the charges incurred in moving the grounded boat off public property.

18

Watkins sloop, 27 feet, 7,500 pounds displacement, 3 feet 8 inches draft, aground on a rocky Penobscot Bay, Maine, peninsula.

The cruising sailboat had been grounded near high tide because of a piloting error. Attempts at kedging had failed to move the vessel, essentially because of a rapid increase in the depth of water in the direction of the desired pull. The downward angle of the kedge line forced the keel down. The skipper, reasoning that a horizontal pull would free the keel, hailed a passing 35-foot cruising sailboat. The assisting boat dropped its anchor in deep water, backed down the full length of available rode (about 325 feet) to a point near the disabled boat, and transferred a towline. Once the towline was secured properly, the assisting boat used its hydraulic anchor winch to put a strain on the towline, while the disabled craft's crew heeled their boat by placing two crewmembers on the end of the swung-out boom. The boat moved off easily into deep water, the strong horizontal tow preventing the unpleasant necessity of drying out in the 9-foot tidal range.

19

Albin trawler, 36 feet, 18,500 pounds displacement, 3 foot 6 inches draft, tanks: fuel 350 gallons/water 220 gallons, aground on Florida sand beach.

The power yacht was forced aground on a lee shore by Hurricane David, which had 70-m.p.h. winds at Fort Pierce, gusting to 95 m.p.h. The large bow anchor was dropped before the trawler went aground, but, used as a kedge, it was unable to move the boat. The crew of three made it safely ashore through the rampaging high surf, taking with them two shore lines to keep the boat from moving about excessively. The sturdy boat was not damaged, and the crew expected her to survive the fast-moving storm. As the majority of the waves struck the vessel broadside, with quieter waters at the bow and stern, a sandbar quickly formed amidships. Soon the craft was supported only by the sandbar, as the surf scoured material from the forward and aft sections, breaking the back of the cruiser. The tanks filled with about 3,500 pounds of fuel and water contributed to the problem. The boat was a total loss. The case is identical to that of many stranded ships that have been lost because of this phenomenon, known as a *tombolo*.

20

O'Day sloop, 23 feet, 3,725 pounds displacement, 2 feet 3 inches draft, aground on rock shore of a Boston Harbor island.

The popular-sized sailboat was reported stolen from its Inner Harbor marina slip and discovered high aground the next day by the city Harbor Patrol. Apparently the boat had been grounded at high water during a spring tide, for the boat was high and dry during ensuing high tides, only 20 feet inland but 12 feet above the water on a rock ledge. The owners, two young MIT engineering students, decided to devise their own portable crane apparatus to lift the boat off its high rock perch and swing it back into the sea. After calculating the material strength requirements necessary to lift the sloop, they visited several Boston-area metal salvage yards to look for the material to build a crane. They purchased a sizable, but inexpensive, quantity of scrap aluminum building girders, with the promise of a refund if the same amount of aluminum was returned to the yard when the job was completed. Scrap elevator cable was also obtained the same way, and the students designed and prefabricated a crane. The light material was cut to a manageable size, to be bolted together later at the scene of the stranding. They borrowed the yacht club launch to transport the girders, together with a cumbersome, but powerful, hand-cranked winch. Fellow students volunteered to help, and they spent four hours bolting together the strange-looking apparatus. Then they hoisted the sloop and swung her back into the water. It was a clever and neat exercise in elementary engineering, and the cost was minimal.

21

Catalina sloop, 30 feet, 10,200 pounds displacement, 4 feet 4 inches draft, aground on a remote Southern California beach.

The yacht was caught off a lee shore by a fast-moving gale and, after three hours of barely being able to stand off, was hurled far onto the beach, well beyond the normal shoreline, by a towering wave. Two of the three persons on board were injured. The tide ebbed, leaving the slightly damaged boat high and dry, 140 feet from the water. At high tide, the boat was 65 feet from the water, lying on her starboard side, mast pointing toward the adjacent high cliffs. The crew and the people who assisted in their rescue saw no hope for moving the vessel back into the water immediately, so they departed to seek medical aid and commercial salvage assistance, leaving the boat unattended. That evening, another gale, more vicious than the one that had put the sloop aground, blew onto the coast. Observers high on the cliff road were amazed to see the water rise to surround the disabled boat and then, with one huge wave, pick up the boat and take her seaward. There being no set anchor or shore lines to hold her, she wallowed in the turbulent sea, fending for herself. The seas took her almost one mile southward before an onslaught of waves tossed her aground on a rocky beach, destroying the once-proud vessel.

22

Dickerson sloop, 36 feet, 12,000 pounds displacement, 4 feet draft, aground on a rocky Maine coast

Two couples, experienced in sailing the Maine coast, became disoriented in a thick fog off Petit Manan Point and struck a small submerged ledge island, jamming the full-keeled boat hard aground at high water. They knew from soundings that once the 12-foot tide went down, the yacht would probably settle deeply by the stern, flooding the aft section of the boat. The weather was building from the northeast, the first sign of an expected gale. They reasoned that they would have to refloat the sailboat immediately if they were to save her. They notified the Coast Guard station at Jonesport, 25 miles east, and received an ETA of 75 minutes. This would be too late, as the tide was about to start to ebb, so it was decided to lighten the vessel in an attempt to kedge off. While the crewmembers set the kedge, one rowing out with the 44-pound Bruce anchor while one fed out line from the stern, the skipper opened the diesel-fuel and water-tank lines and pumped 100 gallons of liquid (the boat had a reserve 40-gallon tank) overboard with the bilge pump. Three spare anchors were lowered on lines over the sides. Tools, spare parts, canned goods, and many other heavy items were placed in sail bags and also lowered over the sides of the boat on lines, to be retrieved later. With the engine idling, both large marine batteries were lowered quickly into the dinghy. Bags of sails, clothing, extra radios, charts, and other items were tossed into the dinghy, until it was almost in danger of sinking. Other items, such as books and spare cans of oil, were simply thrown overboard. Even the 50-pound block of ice in the icebox, as well as other contents, was heaved overboard. The kedge line was taken forward to the electric anchor winch and full strain was applied, the engine full throttle in reverse. She didn't move. When the crew was ordered to the stern rail, the sloop slid off the rocks, with only a grinding sound as a sign of protest.

23

Pearson sloop, 30 feet, 8,400 pounds displacement, 5 feet draft, grounded on sand bottom off southern Cape Cod on Nantucket Bay, in mild July weather.

Shortly after the grounding, which was a half mile from shore, the weather quickly deteriorated, with the waves building from 1 foot to about 4 feet on an ebbing tide. The crew of two attempted to deploy a kedge with the dinghy, but they aborted the effort when the dinghy was swamped; the kedge was let go near the disabled boat. Squally winds drove the boat toward shore, dragging her anchor for some distance, the keel pounding on the bottom with each wave. The couple hoisted the sails, ran the engine hard, cast off the kedge line (buoyed, to be retrieved later), and set a course diagonal to the shoreline. They reasoned that the force of the building wind on the sails might heel the boat sufficiently to free the keel. The yacht pounded on the bottom in the wave troughs, but she made headway, gradually breaking free completely and taking them into open water.

24

Irwin Competition sloop, 30 feet, 7,300 pounds displacement, 3 feet 6 inches draft (6 feet 6 inches, centerboard down), aground on a Texas sand shore.

Five racing sailors had been on a downwind run near a long, flat beach when the steering gear failed. The boat was driven hard aground at mid-flood tide. But even when the tide was at full high, they were unable to kedge the boat off the flat beach, where a crowd of perhaps 150 curious observers had formed to see the "shipwreck." A spring tide had occurred two days earlier, so the crew would have to wait about two weeks for another one. To drag the expensive yacht any distance over the relatively flat bottom would surely damage the keel, or worse. If keelbolts sheared during such an ungrounding attempt, the captain reasoned, the keel could be sent through the hull, creating a serious problem of reconstruction. At low tide the yacht lay on her side. Fortunately, the weather was warm and the seas calm. Surf conditions were insignificant, but were known to change quickly. After making several phone calls from a nearby beach house, the skipper returned to the scene and ordered the crew to begin unloading all gear on the beach and to pump the water tanks dry. One crewmember was dispatched by taxi to the local truck-rental garage. Within two hours, a huge truck-mounted crane appeared on the road adjacent to the beach, soon to be joined by a marina tractor with a flatbed boat trailer. The gear was loaded on the rented truck as the crane was brought into position on the beach at low tide. Soon straps were slung under the unfortunate vessel and she was hoisted off the beach and swung 180 degrees to the waiting boat trailer. In short order, the crew climbed aboard the truck and the entire convoy departed for the marina.

25

Benteau Evasion motorsailer, 32 feet, 12,600 pounds displacement, 4 feet 6 inches draft, aground on a Caribbean island shore.

With a crew of three, a couple and a young man, the cruising sailboat had been grounded parallel to the shore on a hard sand and coral bottom. The boat had been operating under power and sail at the time of the grounding. Kedging had failed to move the vessel. Commercial towing services were almost 200 miles away. Other ungrounding techniques had been tried (careening, lightening ship, etc.) on three successive high tides without success. Buoyancy tanks were investigated, but only oil drums were found, and no appropriate air compressor could be secured. They were running out of options when, on a trip to the town, the motorsailer skipper noticed a number of men using long ropes to drag a large fishing boat up on the beach for repairs. Why not use manpower to free the grounded boat? He entered into negotiations with the men pulling the fishing boat, which was partially controlled by the fishing-boat skipper. They, and others, would be at the side of the grounded pleasure boat just after low tide the next day. The motorsailer skipper rigged a hull bridle and several long towlines before 25 men arrived in several old trucks. Chest deep in the water, the men hauled on two large ropes slung over their shoulders, and, aided with a winch on the kedge, they dragged the yacht into deeper water. The very reasonable charge was supplemented with mugs of grog all around.

26

Morgan Out Island sloop, 41 feet, 24,000 pounds displacement, 4 feet 2 inches draft, aground on a Bahamas sand shoal.

Put aground at high tide while motorsailing, the crew of six had tried kedging, careening, and towing to refloat the boat, but still she remained hard aground at both of the following high tides. An underwater examination of the keel revealed that additional sand had piled up against the keel, presumably from local currents. A serious effort to lighten the boat had not appreciably reduced draft requirements. The crew evacuated the stranded boat, in an 11-foot Boston Whaler tender, leaving the skipper aboard on watch. The crew, seeking professional salvage assistance, was unsuccessful because of the remote location of the grounding and the shallowness of the water, which would not allow larger salvage vessels to approach the sailboat. But one of the crew had a different proposal. Why not dredge around the keel and dredge a trench to deep water? It was fast becoming their last hope, so they began to look for a small dredging boat equipped with relatively long suction hoses. Two days later, such a dredge was located, and an agreement was made with the private construction company that owned it. At low tide, the dredge was positioned as close as possible to the stranded yacht. The trench was created in a straight line toward the sailboat, the course being marked by small buoys (plastic containers) moored to the bottom with weights. As the channel was dug, the small dredge scow was winched up the channel on set anchors. The distance was about 250 feet, but the sand that had to be moved (it was pumped via a discharge hose about 100 feet to one side) was only a few inches deep. By the time high tide approached, the extended suction hose had reached the boat and was removing sand from around the keel, with people in the water and in the tender controlling the intake nozzle. The stranded boat soon was kedged off.

27

**Santana sloop, 37 feet, 25,000 pounds
displacement, 5 feet 7 inches draft,
aground in Puget Sound on mud bottom.**

The crew of seven had been racing the sailboat under full sail when driven hard aground into the mud flat near high tide. A kedge was run out quickly toward deeper water, but strain on the line failed to budge the heavy boat. A nearby marina towboat was summoned on the VHF radio, but the tow also failed to break the suction of the mud from the keel. The captain of the disabled boat assembled all the crew on the port side of the boat, telling them of a plan to sally the vessel. The idea was that the combined weight of the crew moving quickly from port to starboard, while the powerboat towed from the stern, might move the keel sufficiently to break the grip of the mud. A practice run was made to determine the best place on each side for them to assemble, and then, on the skipper's whistle command, the seven-man crew dashed first to starboard and then back to the port side. The powerboat put on full power and, after sallying was done eight or ten times, the keel was freed enough to allow the rig to be slid into deeper water. They soon were on their way, thanks to a refloating trick used by sailing-ship masters for more than a century.

28

**Pearson Ensign sloop, 22 feet, 3,000
pounds displacement, 3 feet draft, aground
on a mud bank in the Ohio River.**

The small-sailboat skipper had miscalculated his location and the river's current, going aground on a mud flat 100 feet from the bank. Alone at the time of the incident, he could easily have waded ashore. He carried his 13-pound Danforth anchor as far as he could walk toward deep water and set it, but he could not winch the boat off. She showed signs of moving when he heeled her by hiking out on one side, but then he could not operate the winch, which was pulling the kedge line. Unwilling to leave the boat unattended, he waited, hoping that the wake of a passing tug on this busy river might lift the boat just enough so she could be kedged off. Three hours later, his opportunity came up the river in the form of six barges being pushed by a huge tug. The wash did the trick. As the passing waves lifted and dropped the boat, he winched in on the kedge line, soon floating the boat free.

29

Nicholson center-cockpit ketch, 39 feet, 17,000 pounds displacement, 5 feet 6 inches draft, aground on coral/sand bottom on the Mexican coast.

Driving hard in a 20-knot wind at night, the large cruising sailboat went aground on a high spring tide. A couple and two children were aboard. They were four miles off the coastline, and even at low water, they could see no dry land above the foul bottom. At low tide, the boat would heel 30 degrees to port. The draft had increased considerably from when the boat was underway, since they were running at 6 knots and were heeled 15 to 20 degrees at the time. When the boat went aground, the keel was still at that same angle. Since they knew that a moving boat has somewhat less draft than one stopped dead in the water, they figured that the draft to refloat the boat would be considerably higher than if they had touched bottom while standing. Their attempts to kedge off in the 2-foot tidal range proved fruitless. The Mexican Coast Guard made a tow attempt, but they gave up when they were incapable of moving the grounded sailboat and offered to take the crew to the nearest port. Commercial assistance was not suitable; the only available seagoing crane was mounted on a barge whose draft precluded it from approaching the grounded craft. The only apparent solutions were to attempt to heel the boat slightly more than that when she went aground, or to abandon her where she was. They decided to careen the boat while kedging. Using their six-person life-raft as a barge, they transferred all possible items into the raft to reduce weight. Most of the fresh water and fuel was pumped overboard. Other items were thrown overboard, including 150 books, canned goods, etc. The largest anchor was set 300 feet to port for careening, and a spinnaker halyard was attached to an anchor line, which ran to the kedge. A deck block allowed the line to be led to the hydraulic anchor winch. A bridle was made for the stern kedge, and each leg was taken to a cockpit sheet winch. At extreme high tide, they could move the boat somewhat by careening her to about 30 degrees with the masthead line while kedging. It was hard work: The careening anchor had to be reset repeatedly as the boat was backed out while heeled. They set buoys, weighted to the bottom, to measure their progress, which was sometimes as little as 50 feet on a high tide. In all, it took six high tides to get the ketch into water deep enough to float free, a distance of perhaps 300 feet, but they had saved the boat.

30

Sabre sloop, 28 feet, 6,500 pounds displacement, 4 feet 3 inches draft, aground on mud bottom in the St. Lawrence Seaway, New York side.

Three young, but experienced, sailors drove the modern Maine-built auxiliary sailboat hard aground when motorsailing, allegedly forced off course by a small ship. They tried kedging and careening without notable success. Hard use of the engine churned up the soft mud, clogging the raw-water engine intake hose, which twice had to be removed and cleaned when the engine overheated. A passing 32-foot twin-screw powerboat hailed a tow offer, which was accepted promptly. The powerboat backed down to within 40 feet of the stranded sailboat and transferred the bitter end of a ¾-inch nylon anchor line by hand-thrown messenger line. Two 20-foot legs of a bridle were belayed to the two stern cleats of the sailboat and to the towline with bowlines. The powerboat slowly drew the line taut, then applied full power, the three sailors standing at the stern rail of the sailboat. The port stern cleat pulled out under the tremendous strain of the tow, the stern of the sailboat slammed hard to port, and the disabled boat heeled over hard, her stern low in the water. The rudder jammed on the ground, being twisted and broken beyond immediate repair. The sailboat was ungrounded, but now she was disabled in another way; she had to be hauled out for expensive repairs.

31

Tartan Offshore ketch, 40 feet, 24,500 pounds displacement, 4 feet 10 inches draft, aground on the coral/sand bottom off the Florida shore in the Gulf of Mexico.

The ketch had been caught offshore by Hurricane Frederic while attempting to make a harbor of refuge. Winds to 145 m.p.h. forced the boat ashore as the main track of the hurricane passed to the west, making a landfall on the western Florida panhandle. The crew of four was miraculously saved, but five other small-boat sailors perished in the storm. The August/September hurricane lasted for two weeks before weakening to a mere gale as it crossed Newfoundland. Two days after it passed Florida, however, a salvage attempt was made on the grounded boat. The boat was kept from being driven onto the heavy-surfed shore by a small sand island, flanked by mangrove, and three anchors. She was holed and partially filled with water. The extremely high tide created by the storm had left the boat still 18 inches short of enough water to float at high tide. Sufficient water depth was 75 yards away. The owner, a mechanical engineer who had been a minesweeper engineer during a hitch in the Navy, worked with a commercial salvage company to devise a solution for refloating the boat. The plan was simple and effective. The hull holes were repaired with blocks of wood on the interior and exterior, held tightly together with through-bolts after gaskets were in place. She was pumped dry and all removable weight was taken off, including 150 gallons of fresh water, 75 gallons of diesel fuel, the boom, ground tackle, and so forth. A barge with a crane was brought as close as possible, the reach of the extended crane falling short by 80 feet. A 2-inch towline was taken from the boom of the lowered crane to a hull bridle on the disabled yacht. At high tide, steadied by port and starboard anchor lines, the boat was dragged slowly across the sandy bottom toward the barge. The six lines that held her upright (three on each side) were reset regularly, temporarily halting dragging operations. The heavy-displacement yacht was inched ahead until she was in a position to be lifted out with the hull straps. The barge moved off, thus refloating the boat, which was towed to a local harbor.

32

Custom fiberglass sloop, 28 feet, 7,600 pounds displacement, 6 feet 3 inches draft, aground on a Maine mud flat.

The crew of three had allowed the boat to slip out of the bay channel they were navigating, getting stuck in the soft bottom two hours after high tide. After kedging had failed to extricate her, they knew that the boat would have to dry out as the 12-foot tide dropped. They also knew from past experience that the boat would lie over so far that the cockpit —perhaps even the entire interior—would be flooded with the incoming tide. Two of the crew immediately rowed the dinghy ashore, carrying an axe and a small handsaw from the vessel, to look for logs to make temporary legs for the boat. The crewmember who remained aboard prepared the boat's second anchor for use. After the first log was cut from a tree ashore and towed back to the disabled boat, the rower set the kedge anchor off the port beam and the second anchor off to starboard. These two anchor lines held the boat upright (the boat was still floating) and one pole leg was set on each side of the boat. A third timber was lashed to the tops of these poles, then to the bases of the shrouds and to the mast, forming a rigid structure. A crewmember in the water lashed guylines to the leg bases and to cleats forward and aft on the boat. At low tide, the boat stood upright on her own legs, the keel mired in the mud. At high water, the legs were dismounted and the sloop sailed away.

33

Bertram Convertible powerboat, 46 feet, 45,300 pounds displacement, 4 feet 6 inches draft, aground on mud bank in Baltimore Harbor.

A slight piloting error had put the luxury yacht lightly aground on a falling tide. The owner/operator, not wishing to disrupt the happy excursion that the 18 passengers were enjoying, employed a conventional ungrounding technique in a somewhat unconventional fashion.

He radiotelephoned a harbor tug company with which he was familiar, inquiring if they had or soon would have a tug in the area of the grounding. They responded in the affirmative, stating that their largest tug was shortly expected to pass the powerboat's position. When the powerboat operator was patched through to the tug captain, he requested that the tug make a couple of passes at full throttle near the stranded boat. The tug skipper was delighted to comply. As the huge wash from the wake of the tug struck the powerboat, she was lifted clear of the bottom, and, with engines in full reverse, the boat jerked herself free and backed into deeper water. Some of the passengers never even realized they had been aboard a grounded boat.

34

Hunter sloop, 27 feet, 7,000 pounds displacement, 4 feet 3 inches draft, aground on a New Jersey sand beach.

The boat, for reasons yet undiscovered, had her bow rammed hard onto a remote section of a public beach shortly before high tide. The crew of four (two couples) tried kedging off while heeling the boat, but they could not get sufficient power from the cockpit jibsheet winch to move the boat enough to break free. One of the crew suggested that a block-and-tackle system be attached to the kedge line to obtain additional power. They prepared a four-purchase system made up from Dacron sheets and spare halyards. The kedge was also reset farther out in the direction of deep water. By this time, a small crowd of sunbathers and swimmers had gathered to observe the grounded boat, so 16 bystanders were recruited, in addition to three crewmembers, to haul in on the bitter end of the fall. Amid hoots and hollers, the sloop slid back into the water.

35

Custom wooden yawl, 36 feet, approximately 20,000 pounds displacement, 5 feet 1 inch draft, aground on a British Columbia island shore.

The older yawl had been pounded severely by a massive storm, springing a hull plank, which caused serious flooding. The two-man crew bailed constantly for eight hours, at the same time dealing with the storm, but the inflow of water could not be stemmed, so they decided to beach the boat in an effort to save her. They were unable to go to the protected side of a nearby island, however, and were forced to run her onto a lee beach. Aground in the surf, the boat pounded badly. The crew reasoned that to keep the boat from breaking up and becoming flotsam, they would have to scuttle her. After opening all portholes and hatches, they sank the boat by pulling off two through-hull hoses. When filled, the heavy boat moved little on the bottom. They managed to take ashore long bow and stern lines, which were tied to boulders to keep the boat from moving farther. When the tide receded, the water drained from the hull, allowing them to make temporary hull repairs. One external patching arrangement was held in place with a small-diameter chain, which completely girdled the boat and was held taut with a block-and-tackle arrangement on deck until more permanent repairs could be made. They had managed to save the boat by sinking her and were able to refloat her on the next high tide.

36

Yamaha sloop, 26 feet, 4,400 pounds displacement, 5 feet 1 inch draft, aground on a sharply sloping California beach.

The racing boat went aground shortly after high tide, parallel to the shoreline. As the water receded, the boat heeled seaward. The crew of four was unable to heel the boat shoreward, or to the high side of the sloping bottom, thus placing the hull in danger of flooding as the tide returned. Three crewmembers went ashore immediately to seek shoring to hold the boat from going over completely on the downhill side of the bottom. The owner of a large estate provided them with old planks, which had been stored in the attic of his horse barn. A series of 10 long planks was dug into the bottom at an angle and lashed to the toerail and deck fittings of the boat, holding her at a 30-degree list at low tide. With high tide, the boat floated, no water having entered, and the crew returned the borrowed planks to their owner before departing the scene under sail.

37

Stamas Sport Fisherman, 32 feet, 12,800 pounds displacement, 2 feet 9 inches draft, aground on mud bottom in Charleston, South Carolina, Harbor.

The sturdy, oceangoing powerboat went hard aground on the harbor shore while maneuvering under power through the early stage of Hurricane Dora. The 65-m.p.h. winds were building against the stern of the grounded boat, which was in the direction of deeper water. Eventually they reached 125 m.p.h. The owner/operator knew that the best chance of survival for the boat was to secure her to a large mooring, 300 feet from the stranding. He was unable to obtain commercial or Coast Guard towing assistance because of the fast-moving hurricane, and there was no way that the crew of two could set a kedge, primarily because the small dinghy had been upset twice in the high waves while carrying a heavy anchor. The yacht was pounding badly in the surf, and, if allowed to continue, would surely be broken up. Quickly they launched a 13-foot Boston Whaler from a nearby dock, and, charging through the turbulent harbor, one man took the bitter end of a heavy anchor line out to a ship mooring buoy. He rove it through the eye of the huge steel buoy before beating his way back toward the grounded boat. The man aboard the disabled boat had fed out line, adding a second anchor rode and docklines to bring the total length of line to about 1,000 feet. Once the line was ashore, it was tied to the trailer hitch of a marina truck. The other end was made fast to a stern bridle made up for the sportfisherman. With truck tires squealing, twin 250-h.p. gasoline boat engines in full reverse roared, and the boat thumped off. The tow continued as the line on the truck was tied and untied several times, until the boat was bumping against the ship mooring buoy. As soon as she was belayed to the buoy, the operator took a rollercoaster ride to shore in an inflatable dinghy. The eight-ton mooring held the sportfisherman throughout the storm.

38

Cheoy Lee long-range motorsailer, 43 feet, 34,000 pounds displacement, 5 feet draft, aground on mud bottom in Boston Harbor.

The offshore sailboat, with a crew of five, was completing a successful 2,500-mile voyage from South America when the boat unexpectedly went aground. The navigator had the large boat correctly on course, but he had neglected to calculate properly all the factors affecting tidal levels. It was a perigean spring low, the lowest tide phase of the year. When the crew could not ascertain the cause of the problem, misunderstanding the U.S. chart datums, they fled the craft. Soon a Coast Guard patrol boat appeared, finding the boat loaded with bales of marijuana that police valued at several million dollars. At a higher stage of the tide, the boat floated and was towed to the Harbor Police Wharf. TV news coverage of the grounded boat was extensive, but the reporters failed to mention why she went aground.

39

Tanzer sloop, 24 feet, 3,800 pounds displacement, 4 feet draft, aground on a Lake Erie rocky shore.

The boat was driven hard aground under full sail by her crew of four. Shortly afterward, a 28-foot Uniflite powerboat appeared, offering a tow. The bitter end of a ½-inch-diameter, 250-foot-long nylon anchor rode was passed to the twin-engined powerboat, while the other end was secured to a mid-transom cleat. The powerboat, bow facing the stranded boat, applied full reverse power. The nylon line increased its length by one-third under the heavy strain. The stern cleat parted and went flying, like a bullet, still attached to the line, toward the power-boat. Two people on the foredeck of the powerboat ducked, avoiding the missile by inches. The flying cleat crashed through the windshield, coming to rest at the transom of the powerboat, line still attached. The grounded sailboat crew elected to kedge their boat off the shore. The next cleat they installed was properly backed and bolted.

40

Schock sloop, 30 feet, 6,800 pounds displacement, 5 feet 6 inches draft, aground on a California harbor mud bottom.

The racing sailboat was driven hard aground, while under power, in a crowded marina area with five crewmembers aboard. The crew tried, without success, to refloat the boat with long lines strung to adjacent docks. A 32-foot Trojan Convertible powerboat with twin 270-h.p. gasoline inboard engines, docked nearby, offered to tow the grounded sailboat. The Trojan was able to maneuver into place skillfully in the tight quarters of the marina, her 2½-foot draft allowing for stern-to-stern transfer of a ¾-inch Dacron towline. The line was belayed to a short bridle attached to the sailboat's stern cleats. Large sailboats were docked on both sides of the grounded sailboat, and the Trojan had only 50 feet of clearance ahead. The skipper of the Trojan applied full throttle to his engines, the boats bucked and jumped, and the sail-boat was jerked free. But as the sailboat became ungrounded, the two boats charged ahead, out of control. The Trojan skipper put his helm hard over, forcing the stern of the sloop hard to starboard, causing her to collide violently with an adjacent boat, crazing her hull. A sailboat crewmember was thrown over the lifelines and onto the deck of the adjacent boat, breaking his arm. The collision forced the bow of the sailboat to swing out of control, ramming into yet another boat on her other side, causing more damage. The three separate insurance companies involved in the incident all agreed that towing in tight quarters is tricky business.

41

Bertram Flybridge Cruiser, 28 feet, 10,000 pounds displacement, 2 feet 7 inches draft, powered by twin 233-h.p. gas engines, aground in a Louisiana back waterway.

The powerboat was traveling at a high rate of speed along a remote island waterway when she was run hard and high aground, coming to rest some 100 feet from the waterway, her bottom sustaining a 3-foot-long gash as it was driven against a rock ledge. The two couples aboard were unhurt. They used the VHF radiotelephone to summon assistance and were transported from the scene by a local boat operator. The closest road to the area was almost 10 miles away from the site, and the distance between was swampy in several places. The waterway was of such a width and depth as to exclude a barge large enough to transport the boat. Moreover, the damage to the boat was considered severe enough to preclude temporary patching. After careful evaluation, it was determined that the craft could be lifted off by a helicopter sky crane. A work party traveled by boat to the site, where they used hydraulic jacks to place a hoisting harness around the boat. They cut down several nearby trees to provide for ample swinging room and removed what weight they could from the craft. Long lines were attached forward and aft to guide the lift. At the designated hour, the sky crane hovered over the boat. A cable was shackled to the harness and the boat was lifted off, assisted by men holding the lines. Thirty minutes later, the boat was being guided into a cradle at a marina.

42

Steel-hulled trawler, 87 feet, 153 tons displacement, 6 feet 8 inches draft, aground on a flat, sandy Northern California beach during a spring high tide.

The Oregon-based vessel was forced ashore during a ferocious December storm when she lost her main engine. The combined effects of high tide, high surf, and gale-force winds caused the disabled vessel to drag anchor and end up abnormally high on the beach. Her rudder was broken off at the stock and her propeller and skeg were bent. Luckily, she was high enough to avoid being pounded by the surf. Discussions about refloating the large boat soon focused on the fact that she was built without longitudinals, so it was feared that a conventional tow-off would result in major structural damage. The bids to refloat the $375,000 boat were $35,000 and $31,500, the latter from a house-mover who had 12 years of experience in moving boats on land with hydraulic jacks. The house-mover got the job. The operation, which took seven days, went off without a hitch. First the boat's fuel, water, and heavy gear were offloaded. Then metal plates were welded to the rubrails amidships, port and starboard, in preparation for mounting the hydraulic rams, which were powered by a 10,000-pound pump. To move the boat toward the water, the stern was raised with the rams (long hydraulic cylinders belayed on pivot points vertically against the sides). Sand was excavated from astern with a backhoe, and the bow was pushed straight back with a bulldozer while the rams were lowered, causing the boat to creep in short steps backward toward the water. (The bulldozer was fitted with a special timber fork to push against the bow.) This operation was repeated until the vessel was in a suitable position for towing at high tide. A 1,000-h.p. tug secured a towline to the disabled boat and successfully towed her off for repairs. The salvors maintain that this technique of raising the stern or bow of a boat with long, pivoted hydraulic rams and then pushing the boat in slow stages in the desired direction can be useful in many grounding situations. (For wooden or fiberglass boats, they state, some cosmetic damage would result from mounting the ram plates.) They further found that improvements in the hydraulic ram system could reduce the need for much of the heavy equipment used in the trawler operation, such as moving the boat (once lifted) with strain on a kedge line. The need to remove bottom material might also be eliminated in many cases.

Minimum Rope-Breaking Strength (in pounds)[1]

DIAMETER		TWISTED AND PLAITED ROPES				
Inches	MM	Manila	Polypropylene	Polyester*	Nylon	Prestretched Polyester*
3/16	5	406	720	900	900	1,300
1/4	6	540	1,130	1,490	1,490	1,550
5/16	8	900	1,710	2,300	2,300	3,300
3/8	9	1,220	2,240	3,340	3,340	4,000
7/16	10	1,580	3,160	4,500	4,500	5,000
1/2	12	2,380	3,780	5,750	5,750	6,000
9/16	14	3,100	4,600	7,200	7,200	—
5/8	16	3,960	5,600	9,000	9,350	—
3/4	18	4,860	7,650	11,300	12,800	—
7/8	22	6,950	10,400	16,200	18,000	—
1	24	8,100	12,600	19,800	22,600	—

[1]Cordage Institute figures, which may vary from manufacturer to manufacturer. Safe working loads under normal conditions are typically 20% of each figure given.

Polyester is the generic term used for fibers manufactured under the trademarks of Dacron, Terylene, and Duron.

BRAIDED ROPES

Polyester* Double Braid	Prestretched Polyester*	Nylon Double Braid	Low-Stretch Polyester*
1,000	1,050	—	—
1,800	1,250	2,100	2,200
2,800	2,650	3,500	3,300
3,750	—	4,800	4,400
5,500	4,000	6,500	5,800
7,000	5,000	8,300	8,300
10,000	—	11,200	11,000
14,000	—	14,500	13,600
16,000	—	18,000	—
24,000	—	26,500	—
28,000	—	31,300	—

U.S. Coast Guard Towing and Salvage Policies*

1. **GENERAL TOWING POLICIES:** The area commander or the district commander, upon receipt of information that a vessel or person is disabled or in potential distress, should send a Coast Guard vessel or aircraft, as appropriate, to the scene. Upon arrival at the scene, assistance rendered may include, but is not limited to, the following:
   a. Technical assistance furnished on the spot.
   b. Miscellaneous supplies and equipment furnished for the purpose of effecting temporary repair on the spot.
   c. Towage to the nearest port in which emergency repairs can be made.
      (1) Towing to the nearest port where emergency repairs can be effected does not imply that the port must have complete facilities to perform permanent repair work. Nor does it imply that the Coast Guard should tow the vessel to the repair yard itself. Normally, in a port where commercial towing is available, the Coast Guard will have discharged its responsibility when the distressed vessel is brought to a safe harborage.

*From the Coast Guard Addendum to the *National Search and Rescue Manual.*

(Note: If a vessel is loaded with perishable cargo, a tow to the nearest port where the cargo may be discharged will normally be provided, if the operational situation permits.)

2. **VESSEL OUT OF FUEL:** Many cases arise where the vessel is dis abled because of lack of fuel. The cause of the fuel shortage is immaterial, although in most cases it is poor judgment. In all such cases, a check should be made on arrival at the scene to determine if the vessel does in fact require fuel to reach the nearest port where fuel may be obtained. If a shortage exists, sufficient fuel to reach the nearest port may be invoiced to the vessel. Due regard for weather conditions existing or expected should be exercised. If the Coast Guard vessel does not have the proper fuel, then towage to the nearest fueling port is indicated as outlined below.

3. **COMMERCIAL ENTERPRISE:** Although the Coast Guard will not compete or interfere with private towing activities or other commercial enterprise, it cannot rely upon private enterprise to render assistance in minor cases and itself act only when extreme jeopardy exists. Even though reliable information is received that a tug or other private assistance is proceeding to the scene, there is no assurance that it will complete the mission until it is on scene and has the situation in hand. Until then the Coast Guard units should proceed toward the scene.

   a. If, upon arrival at the scene, private enterprise is already there and is rendering assistance, or is willing to render assistance, the Coast Guard shall not interfere with the private activity unless it becomes apparent that private enterprise cannot cope with the situation and that action by the Coast Guard is necessary to prevent loss of life or property. The private salvor's ability to carry out the operation is best determined by the Coast Guard on-scene commander, but if doubt exists, the matter may be referred to the district commander. (Note: In all doubtful cases, however, the Coast Guard unit shall stand by and be prepared to render assistance until it is apparent that no further assistance is required.)

   b. When the Coast Guard unit is already rendering assistance and private assistance arrives on-scene, the Coast Guard vessel shall turn the case over to the private operator if:

   (1) He desires to accept it.

   (2) The character of the assistance he can render is adequate.

   (3) The operator of the assisted vessel agrees.

   (4) The shift of responsibility can be accomplished without further endangering the craft in trouble. (Note: Actual refusal to

release the disabled vessel to a private operator whose facilities are deemed inadequate will only be done after careful consideration.)

c. Should the operator of this disabled vessel, or the owner of an unmanned vessel, refuse to accept commercial assistance, or remain silent, the Coast Guard will discontinue towing and stand by. Caution: This step will only be taken if the disabled vessel is not further endangered. Otherwise the tow shall be continued until it can be discontinued without danger.

d. If towing to the vicinity of a harbor entrance or safe anchorage under these circumstances, the possibility of the towed vessel creating a hazard should be carefully considered. The length of time that a Coast Guard vessel is required to stand by while the commercial salvor and disabled vessel are negotiating will depend on the circumstances. Should a more urgent case arise, the Coast Guard is free to depart and undertake the more urgent case.

e. If no other cases are pending, the Coast Guard vessel should stand by until negotiations are concluded, and the commercial salvor has taken the disabled vessel in tow. Should a Coast Guard vessel arrive at the scene before a commercial salvage vessel, the Coast Guard vessel may take the vessel in tow pending arrival of the salvage vessel, if such action will contribute to the safety of the distressed vessel or reduce the time in which the Coast Guard vessel is required to stand by.

4. **GENERAL SALVAGE POLICY (OTHER THAN TOWING):** Coast Guard units should engage in salvage other than towing only when no commercial salvage facilities are on scene performing salvage, and limited salvage operations (e.g., ungrounding, pumping, damage control measures, etc.) by the Coast Guard can prevent a worsening situation or complete loss of the vessel. When commercial salvors are on scene performing salvage, Coast Guard units may assist them within the unit's capabilities, if the salvor requests. Coast Guard units and personnel shall not be unduly hazarded in performing salvage under the authority of this section.

5. **TOWING AND SALVAGE OF SMALL CRAFT:** Conflicts relative to towing and salvage of large vessels seldom arise since arrangements are usually made between the owners or agents and private salvage companies. With smaller boats and vessels, the value of property is such that private towing is often unprofitable. In such cases the Coast Guard unit may be the only one in position to render assistance. Even should private towing assistance be of-

fered, the operator of a small craft is under no obligation to accept it. Should he refuse, a Coast Guard unit is not obliged to assist as long as the private towing vessel is standing by. If it departs or if the situation worsens to the extent that life or property are in danger, the Coast Guard unit then should render assistance.

a. SECTION B (5) applies to small craft which need salvage other than towing. However, when no commercial salvage companies are available within a reasonable time or distance, the district commander may modify the policy of SECTION B (5) to provide for refloating a grounded boat which is not in peril of further damage or loss, providing:

   (1) The Coast Guard units are capable of rendering assistance.

   (2) The owner requests the assistance and agrees to the specific effort to be made.

   (3) Coast Guard units and personnel are not unduly hazarded by the operation. *Warning:* Occasionally an operator will insist that the Coast Guard take action, such as pulling a vessel from a reef, that the Coast Guard personnel on scene consider unwise. The Coast Guard is under no obligation to agree to any such request or demand. If a decision to comply with such a request is made, it should be made clear to the operator that he/she is assuming the risk of the operation and the fact that the action is undertaken at his/her request against our advice should be logged.

6. **GENERAL PROCEDURES WHEN TOWING VESSELS UNDER 65 FEET IN LENGTH:**

   a. Wearing of personal flotation devices (PFD): Towing Is a potentially dangerous evolution, which is often compounded by poor weather conditions and the crossing of breaking bars or inlets. While every effort is made to insure the safety of life and property in all instances, the fact remains that a number of boats each year sink or capsize while under tow by the Coast Guard. Occasionally, loss of life has resulted from these mishaps. Since the wearing of personal flotation devices would reduce the possibility of loss of life during towing operations, vessels under sixty-five (65) feet should normally not be taken in tow until all persons on board the towed vessel are wearing approved personal flotation devices. While it is recognized that every towing situation does not warrant the wearing of PFDs, it must be remembered that the safety of the POB (people on board) and the vessel being towed is in part the responsibility of the boat coxswain and the Coast Guard; therefore, the wearing of PFDs must at least be considered in every towing evolution. In cases where insufficient personal flotation devices are available, Coast Guard personal flotation devices, in excess of crew requirements on the assisting unit(s), should be furnished for those persons in need of them. Caution: At no time should the stricken vessel be left in immediate danger while waiting for personnel aboard to don their personal flotation devices.

b. If there are insufficient personal flotation devices to go around, do not wait for more to arrive before rendering assistance. Priority consideration upon arriving at the distress scene is:

(1) Removing the vessel and occupants from immediate danger.

(2) Getting all personnel into personal flotation devices as soon as possible. Caution: It is stressed that only wearable types of personal flotation devices fully meeting safety requirements are used; however, other types may be used if not enough wearable PFDs are available.

c. Removal of Personnel: When conditions warrant and the opportunity is presented, it is desirable to remove all civilians from a disabled craft, and place a Coast Guardman aboard. This decision should be made only with the concurrence of the people involved. The determining factor should be the safety of the people and the boat involved, considering the hazards of going alongside. Prudence should be exercised to avoid making a bad situation worse. Consideration should be given to the weather conditions and the design of vessel, as well as the physical and psychological state of the POB.

d. Deck Fittings: Another hazard in towing small craft involves the poor strength characteristics of cleats and fittings aboard many of today's pleasure craft. Caution: Extreme caution should be used in determining the best possible towing procedure and methods of attaching the towline. The stem pad-eye which is available on most trailerized small boats may be an appropriate point of attachment, however, a close inspection of the condition of the pad-eye, the apparent condition of the stem, and the pad-eye backing plate and nut should be accomplished before selecting the stem pad-eye as the point to attach the towline. Age of fitting, size of fitting, boat loading, sea conditions, towing course relative to sea/swell may all be factors which would make the stem pad-eye a poor attachment point for the towline.

e. Communications: Under certain operating conditions involving the towing evolution, it is essential that a system of communication with the towed vessel be established. The coxswain of the towing boat must insure that those he is assisting understand and agree on a signal to indicate trouble. Ideally, stationing a Coast Guardman on board with a portable communication rig would insure quick response to urgent situations. As an alternative, most units have portable radios that could be carried on board Coast Guard boats when underway, thereby providing a ready communication resource which could be transferred to the disabled vessel utilizing some type of watertight enclosure. Directions for use of the radio are on the back of the set. However, the radio could be switched on and preset for working frequency, prior to transfer to the disabled vessel in order to insure immediate operation. This procedure would be of particular value during night-time operations. Other methods such as flashing lights, warning flag or rag, hand signals, etc., may also be utilized by the coxswain, depending on the on-scene conditions. (Note: It must be remembered that it is incumbent on Coast Guard personnel to learn as much as possible about conditions on the towed vessel, and this information must be continuously updated. Regular checks utilizing the radio or other means of communication are essential elements which will assist in insuring a safe evolution.)

f. Tidal Considerations: Many of the incidents which resulted in damage to grounded small craft could have been avoided by waiting for a rising tide before attempting to refloat, and by inspecting the hull in some manner to determine if it is watertight. The fact that certain small craft are left high and dry by receding tide may not cause damage, if suitable preventer lines are rigged to prevent capsizing, or to maintain it upright on the incoming tide.

g. Liability Releases: The question has often been raised as to the need for Coast Guard units to obtain a liability release prior to rendering aid. Court decisions do not generally favor the use of releases to avoid liability for future negligence, especially in situations where the person giving the release is in an emergency situation and has little choice in the matter. (Note: Coast Guard personnel should concentrate on the primary task of assisting persons and property in danger to the best of their ability, realizing that the best defense against any allegation of negligence is to be able to show that a high standard of care was exercised when rendering assistance. Liability releases shall not be used in assistance cases.)

Lloyd's Standard Form of Salvage Agreement, No Cure—No Pay

On board the _____

Dated _____ 19____

IT IS HEREBY AGREED between Captain[1] _____ for and on behalf of the Owners of the "_____" her Cargo and Freight and _____ for and on behalf of _____ (hereinafter called "the Contractor")[2]:

1. The Contractor agrees to use his best endeavours to salve the _____ and her cargo and take them unto _____ or other place to be hereafter agreed with the Master, providing at his own risk all proper steam and other assistance and labour. The ser-

[1] Insert name of person signing on behalf of owners of property to be salved.

[2] The Contractor's name should always be inserted in line 3 and whenever the Agreement is signed by the Master of the Salving vessel or other person on behalf of the Contractor the name of the Master or other person must also be inserted in line 3 before the words "for and on behalf of". The words "for and on behalf of" should be deleted where a Contractor signs personally.

vices shall be rendered and accepted as salvage services upon the principle of "no cure—no pay" and the Contractor's remuneration in the event of success shall be[3] _____, unless this sum shall afterwards be objected to as hereinafter mentioned in which case the remuneration for the services rendered shall be fixed by Arbitration in London in the manner hereinafter prescribed: and any other difference arising out of this Agreement or the operations thereunder shall be referred to Arbitration in the same way. In the event of the services referred to in this Agreement or any part of such services having been already rendered at the date of this Agreement by the Contractor to the said vessel or her cargo it is agreed that the provisions of this Agreement shall mutatis mutandis apply to such services.

2. The Contractor may make reasonable use of the vessel's gear anchors and chains and other appurtenances during and for the purpose of the operations free of costs but shall not unnecessarily damage abandon or sacrifice the same or any other of the property.

3. Notwithstanding anything hereinbefore contained should the operations be only partially successful without any negligence or want of ordinary skill and care on the part of the Contractor or of any person by him employed in the operations, and any portion of the Vessel's Cargo or Stores be salved by the Contractor, he shall be entitled to reasonable remuneration not exceeding a sum equal to _____ per cent of the estimated value of the property salved at _____ or if the property salved shall be sold there then not exceeding the like percentage of the net proceeds of such sale after deducting all expenses and customs duties or other imposts paid or incurred thereon but he shall not be entitled to any further remuneration reimbursement or compensation whatsoever and such reasonable remuneration shall be fixed in case of difference by Arbitration in manner hereinafter prescribed.

4. The Contractor shall immediately after the termination of the services or sooner notify the Committee of Lloyd's of the amount for which he requires security to be given; and failing any such notification by him not later than 48 hours (exclusive of Sundays or other days observed as general holidays at Lloyd's) after the termination of the services he shall be deemed to require security to be given for the sum

---

[3]If at the time of the signing of this Agreement it is not possible to decide upon the figure to be inserted in Clause 1 the space may be left blank as the question of security is dealt with in Clause 4 and the Form provides for the amount of remuneration, if any, to be decided either by agreement or by Arbitration.

named in Clause 1, or, if no sum be named in Clause 1, then for such sum as the Committee of Lloyd's in their absolute discretion shall consider sufficient. Such security shall be given in such manner and form as the Committee of Lloyd's in their absolute discretion may consider sufficient but the Committee of Lloyd's shall not be in any way responsible for the sufficiency (whether in amount or otherwise) of any security accepted by them nor for the default or insolvency of any person firm or corporation giving the same.

5. Pending the completion of the security as aforesaid, the Contractor shall have a maritime lien on the property salved for his remuneration. The salved property shall not without the consent in writing of the Contractor be removed from _____ or the place of safety to which the property is taken by the Contractor on the completion of the salvage services until security has been given to the Committee of Lloyd's as aforesaid. The Contractor agrees not to arrest or detain the property salved unless the security be not given within 14 days (exclusive of Sundays or other days observed as general holidays at Lloyd's) of the termination of the services (the Committee of Lloyd's not being responsibile for the failure of the parties concerned to provide the required security within the said 14 days) or the Contractor has reason to believe that the removal of the property salved is contemplated contrary to the above agreement. In the event of security not being provided as aforesaid or in the event of any attempt being made to remove the property salved contrary to this Agreement the Contractor may take steps to enforce his aforesaid lien. The Arbitrator or Arbitrators or Umpire (including the Committee of Lloyd's if they act in either capacity) appointed under Clause 7 or 8 hereof shall have power in their absolute discretion to include in the amount awarded to the Contractor the whole or such part of the expenses incurred by the Contractor in enforcing his lien as they shall think fit.

6. After the expiry of 42 days from the date of the completion of the security the Committee of Lloyd's shall call upon the party or parties concerned to pay the amount thereof and in the event of non-payment shall realize or enforce the security and pay over the amount thereof to the Contractor unless they shall meanwhile have received written notice of objection and a claim for Arbitration from any of the parties entitled and authorized to make such objection and claim or unless they shall themselves think fit to object and demand Arbitration. The receipt of the Contractor shall be a good discharge to the Committee of Lloyd's for any moneys so paid and they shall incur no

responsibility to any of the parties concerned by making such payment and no objection or claim for Arbitration shall be entertained or acted upon unless received by the Committee of Lloyd's within the 42 days above mentioned.

7. In case of objection being made and Arbitration demanded the remuneration for the services shall be fixed by the Committee of Lloyd's as Arbitrators or at their option by an Arbitrator to be appointed by them unless they shall within 30 days from the date of this Agreement receive from the Contractor a written or telegraphic notice appointing an Arbitrator on his behalf in which case such notice shall be communicated by them to the Owners of the vessel and they shall within 15 days from the receipt thereof give a written notice to the Committee of Lloyd's appointing another Arbitrator on behalf of all the parties interested in the property salved; and if the Owners shall fail to appoint an Arbitrator as aforesaid the Committee of Lloyd's shall appoint an Arbitrator on behalf of all the parties interested in the property salved or they may if they think fit direct that the Contractor's nominee shall act as sole Arbitrator; and thereupon the Arbitration shall be held in London by the Arbitrators or Arbitrator so appointed. If the Arbitrators cannot agree they shall forthwith notify the Committee of Lloyd's who shall thereupon either themselves act as Umpires or shall appoint some other person as Umpire. Any award of the Arbitrators or Arbitrator or Umpire shall (subject to appeal as provided in this Agreement) be final and binding on all the parties concerned and they or he shall have power to obtain call for receive and act upon any such oral or documentary evidence or information (whether the same be strictly admissible as evidence or not) as they or he may think fit, and to conduct the Arbitration in such manner in all respects as they or he may think fit, and to maintain reduce or increase the sum, if any, named in Clause 1, and shall if in their or his opinion the amount of the security demanded is excessive have power in their or his absolute discretion to condemn the Contractor in the whole or part of the expense of providing such security and to deduct the amount in which the Contractor is so condemned from the salvage remuneration. Unless the Arbitrators or Arbitrator or Umpire shall otherwise direct the parties shall be at liberty to adduce expert evidence on the Arbitration. The Arbitrators or Arbitrator and the Umpire (including the Committee of Lloyd's if they act in either capacity) may charge such fees as they may think reasonable, and the Committee of Lloyd's may in any event charge a reasonable fee for their services in connection with the Arbitration, and all such fees shall be treated as part of the

costs of the Arbitration and Award and shall be paid by such of the parties as the Award may direct. Interest at the rate of 5 per cent per annum from the expiration of 14 days (exclusive of Sundays or other days observed as general holidays at Lloyd's) after the date of the publication of the Award by the Committee of Lloyd's until the date of payment to the Committee of Lloyd's shall (subject to appeal as provided in this Agreement) be payable to the Contractor upon the amount of any sum awarded after deduction of any sums paid on account. Save as aforesaid the statutory provisions as to Arbitration for the time being in force in England shall apply. The said Arbitration is hereinafter in this Agreement referred to as "the original Arbitration" and "the Arbitrator or Arbitrators" or "the Umpire" and the Award of such Arbitrator or Arbitrators or Umpire as "the original Award".

8. Any of the persons named under Clause 14, except the Committee of Lloyd's, may appeal from the original Award by giving written Notice of Appeal to the Committee of Lloyd's within 14 days (exclusive of Sundays or other days observed as general holidays at Lloyd's) from the publication by the Committee of Lloyd's of the original Award; and any of the other persons named under Clause 14, except the Committee of Lloyd's, may (without prejudice to their right of appeal under the first part of this clause) within 7 days (exclusive of Sundays or other days observed as general holidays at Lloyd's) after receipt by them from the Committee of Lloyd's of notice of such appeal (such notice if sent by post to be deemed to be received on the day following that on which the said notice was posted) give written Notice of Cross-Appeal to the Committee of Lloyd's. As soon as practicable after receipt of such notice or notices the Committee of Lloyd's shall themselves alone or jointly with another person or other persons appointed by them (unless they be the objectors) hear and determine the Appeal or if they shall see fit to do so or if they be the objectors they shall refer the Appeal to the hearing and determination of a person or persons selected by them. Any Award on Appeal shall be final and binding on all the parties concerned. No evidence other than the documents put in on the original Arbitration and the original Arbitrator's or original Arbitrators' and/or Umpire's notes and/or shorthand notes if any of the proceedings and oral evidence if any at the original Arbitration shall be used on the Appeal unless the Arbitrator or Arbitrators on the Appeal shall in his or their discretion call for other evidence. The Arbitrator or Arbitrators on the Appeal may conduct the Arbitration on Appeal in such manner in all respects as he or they may think fit

and may maintain increase or reduce the sum awarded by the original Award with the like power as is conferred by Clause 7 on the original Arbitrator or Arbitrators or Umpire to condemn the Contractor in the whole or part of the expense of providing security and to deduct the amount disallowed from the salvage remuneration. And he or they shall also make such order as he or they may think fit as to the payment of interest (at the rate of 5 percent per annum) on the sum awarded to the Contractor. The Arbitrator or Arbitrators on Appeal (including the Committee of Lloyd's if they act in that capacity) may direct in what manner the costs of the original Arbitration and of the Arbitration on Appeal shall be borne and paid and may charge such fees as he or they may think reasonable and the Committee of Lloyd's may in any event charge a reasonable fee for their services in connection with the Arbitration on Appeal and all such fees shall be treated as part of the costs of the Arbitration and Award on Appeal and shall be paid by such of the parties as the Award on Appeal shall direct. Save as aforesaid the statutory provisions as to Arbitration for the time being in force in England shall apply.

9. (a) In case of Arbitration if no notice of Appeal be received by the Committee of Lloyd's within 14 days after the publication by the Committee of the original Award the Committee shall call upon the party or parties concerned to pay the amount awarded and in the event of non-payment shall realize or enforce the security and pay therefrom to the Contractor (whose receipt shall be a good discharge to them) the amount awarded to him together with interest as hereinbefore provided.

(b) If notice of Appeal be received by the Committee of Lloyd's in accordance with the provisions of Clause 8 hereof they shall as soon as but not until the Award on Appeal has been published by them, call upon the party or parties concerned to pay the amount awarded and in the event of non-payment shall realize or enforce the security and pay therefrom to the Contractor (whose receipt shall be a good discharge to them) the amount awarded to him together with interest if any in such manner as shall comply with the provisions of the Award on Appeal.

(c) If the Award on Appeal provides that the costs of the original Arbitration or of the Arbitration on Appeal or any part of such costs shall be borne by the Contractor, such costs may be deducted from the amount awarded before payment is made to the Contractor by the Committee of Lloyd's, unless satisfactory security is provided by the Contractor for the payment of such costs.

(d) Without prejudice to the provisions of Clause 4 hereof, the liability of the Committee of Lloyd's shall be limited in any event to the amount of security held by them.

10. The Committee of Lloyd's may in their discretion out of the security (which they may realize or enforce for that purpose) pay to the Contractor on account before the publication of the original Award and/or of the Award on Appeal such sum as they may think reasonable on account of any out-of-pocket expenses incurred by him in connection with the services.

11. The Master or other person signing this Agreement on behalf of the property to be salved is not authorized to make or give and the Contractor shall not demand or take any payment draft or order for or on account of the remuneration.

12. Any dispute between any of the parties interested in the property salved as to the proportions in which they are to provide the security or contribute to the sum awarded or as to any other such matter shall be referred to and determined by the Committee of Lloyd's or by some other person or persons appointed by the Committee whose decision shall be final and is to be complied with forthwith.

13. The Master or other person signing this agreement on behalf of the property to be salved enters into this Agreement as Agent for the vessel her cargo and freight and the respective owners thereof and binds each (but not the one for the other or himself personally) to the due performance thereof.

14. Any of the following parties may object to the sum named in Clause 1 as excessive or insufficient having regard to the services which proved to be necessary in performing the Agreement or to the value of the property salved at the completion of the operations and may claim Arbitration viz: (1) The Owners of the ship. (2) Such other persons together interested as Owners and/or Underwriters of any part not being less than one-fourth of the estimated value of the property salved as the Committee of Lloyd's in their absolute discretion may by reason of the substantial character of their interest or otherwise authorize to object. (3) The Contractor. (4) The Committee of Lloyd's —Any such objection and the original Award upon the Arbitration

following thereon shall (subject to appeal as provided in this Agreement) be binding not only upon the objectors but upon all concerned, provided always that the Arbitrators or Arbitrator or Umpire may in case of objection by some only of the parties interested order the costs to be paid by the objectors only, provided also that if the Committee of Lloyd's be objectors they shall not themselves act as Arbitrators or Umpires.

15. If the parties to any such Arbitration or any of them desire to be heard or to adduce evidence at the original Arbitration they shall give notice to that effect to the Committee of Lloyd's and shall respectively nominate a person in the United Kingdom to represent them for all the purposes of Arbitration and failing such notice and nomination being given the Arbitrators or Arbitrator or Umpire may proceed as if the parties failing to give the same had renounced their right to be heard or adduce evidence.

16. Any Award, notice, authority, order, or other document signed by the Chairman of Lloyd's or a Clerk to the Committee of Lloyd's on behalf of the Committee of Lloyd's shall be deemed to have been duly made or given by the Committee of Lloyd's and shall have the same force and effect in all respects as if it had been signed by every member of the Committee of Lloyd's.

For and on behalf of the
Contractor

For and on behalf of the
Owners of property
to be salved

(To be signed either by the Contractor personally or by the Master of the salving vessel or other person whose name is inserted in line 3 of this Agreement.)

(To be signed by the Master or other person whose name is inserted in line 1 of this Agreement.)

International Code of Signals for Grounding, Beaching, Refloating

Grounding

JF   I am [or vessel indicated is] aground in lat . . . long . . . [also the
following complements, if necessary]:
- 0   On rocky bottom.
- 1   On soft bottom.
- 2   Forward.
- 3   Amidship.
- 4   Aft.
- 5   At high water forward.
- 6   At high water amidship.
- 7   At high water aft.
- 8   Full length of vessel.
- 9   Full length of vessel at high water.

JG   I am aground; I am in dangerous situation.

JH   I am aground; I am not in danger.

       I require immediate assistance; I am aground.   CB 4

       Vessel aground in lat . . . long . . . requires assistance.   C 1

JI   Are you aground?

      JI 1   What was your draft when you went aground?

      JI 2   On what kind of ground have you gone aground?

      JI 3   At what state of tide did you go aground?

      JI 4   What part of your vessel is aground?

JJ   My maximum draft when I went aground was . . . [number] feet or meters.

JK   The tide was high water when the vessel went aground.

      JK 1 The tide was half water when vessel went aground.

      JK 2 The tide was low water when the vessel went aground.

JL   You are running the risk of going aground.

      JL 1 You are running the risk of going aground; do not approach me from the starboard side.

      JL 2 You are running the risk of going aground; do not approach me from the port side.

      JL 3 You are running the risk of going aground; do not approach me from forward.

      JL 4 You are running the risk of going aground; do not approach me from aft.

JM   You are running the risk of going aground at low water.

Beaching

JN   You should beach the vessel in lat . . . long . . .

      JN 1 You should beach the vessel where flag is waved or light is shown.

      JN 2 I must beach the vessel.

Refloating

JO   I am afloat.

      JO 1 I am afloat forward.

      JO 2 I am afloat aft.

      JO 3 I may be got afloat if prompt assistance is given.

      JO 4 Are you [or vessel indicated] still afloat?

JO 5 When do you expect to be afloat?

JP I am jettisoning to refloat [the following complements should be used if required]:
1 Cargo.
2 Bunkers.
3 Everything movable forward.
4 Everything movable aft.

JQ I cannot refloat without jettisoning [the following complements should be used if required]:
1 Cargo.
2 Bunkers.
3 Everything movable forward.
4 Everything movable aft.

JR I expect [or vessel indicated expects] to refloat.
JR 1 I expect [or vessel indicated expects] to refloat at time indicated.
JR 2 I expect [or vessel indicated expects] to refloat in daylight.
JR 3 I expect [or vessel indicated expects] to refloat when tide rises.
JR 4 I expect [or vessel indicated expects] to refloat when visibility improves.
JR 5 I expect [or vessel indicated expects] to refloat when weather moderates.
JR 6 I expect [or vessel indicated expects] to refloat when draft is lightened.
JR 7 I expect [or vessel indicated expects] to refloat when tugs arrive.

JS Is it likely that you [or vessel indicated] will refloat?
JS 1 Is it likely that you [or vessel indicated] will refloat at time indicated?
JS 2 Is it likely that you [or vessel indicated] will refloat in daylight?
JS 3 Is it likely that you [or vessel indicated] will refloat when tide rises?
JS 4 Is it likely that you [or vessel indicated] will refloat when visibility improves?
JS 5 Is it likely that you [or vessel indicated] will refloat when weather moderates?

JS 6 Is it likely that you [or vessel indicated] will refloat when draft is lightened?

JS 7 Is it likely that you [or vessel indicated] will refloat when tugs arrive?

JT I can refloat if an anchor is laid out for me.
JT 1 I may refloat without assistance.
JT 2 Will you assist me to refloat?

JU I cannot be refloated by any means now available.

JV Will you escort me to lat . . . long . . . after refloating?

APPENDIX E

Selected References

Bass, John R. *Marine Salvage: Preservation, Not Possession.* Bar Bulletin, Maine State Bar Association, 1983.

Boat Crew Seamanship Manual. U.S. Coast Guard, 1984.

Boat Handling. Time-Life Books, 1975.

Bowditch, Nathaniel, L.L.D. (original ed.). *American Practical Navigator.* U.S. Navy Hydrographic Office, 1982 edition.

Chapman, Charles F., and Elbert S. Maloney. *Piloting, Seamanship, and Small Boat Handling,* 55th ed. Hearst Marine Books, 1983.

Coles, K. Adlard. *Heavy Weather Sailing.* John de Graff, Inc., 1981.

Gores, Joseph N. *Marine Salvage, The Unforgiving Business of No Cure —No Pay.* Doubleday & Co., 1971.

Hollander, Neil, and Harald Mertes. *The Yachtsman's Emergency Handbook.* Hearst Marine Books, 1980.

LaDage, John, and Lee Van Gemert. *Stability and Trim for the Ship's Officer.* Cornell Maritime Press, 1980.

Lucas, Alan. *The Illustrated Encyclopedia of Boating.* Charles Scribner's Sons, 1977.

Pacific Boating Almanac. Western Marine Enterprises, Inc., published annually.

Parks, Alex L. *The Law of Tug, Tow, and Pilotage,* 2nd ed. Cornell Maritime Press, 1984.

Roth, Hal. *After 50,000 Miles.* W.W. Norton, 1977.

Sanders, R.E. *The Practice of Ocean Rescue.* Brown, Son and Ferguson, Ltd. (Glasgow), 1968.

Ships. Time-Life Books, 1968.

The Visual Encyclopedia of Nautical Terms Under Sail. Crown Publishers, 1978.

U.S. Navy Salvage Manual, Volumes 1–3. Supervisor of Salvage, U.S. Government Printing Office, 1973.

U.S. Navy Salvors Handbook. Supervisor of Salvage, U.S. Navy, U.S. Government Printing Office, 1973.

Waterway Guide, Northern, Mid-Atlantic, Great Lakes, and Southern Editions, published annually.

Wylie, Francis E. *Tides and the Pull of the Moon.* Berkley Books, 1980.

Index